The Bioenergy Story

Michael Yanuck MD PhD

For Bruce, Cynthia, Michael, Paul, Wah, Jennie and Albert.

.

"The most exciting phrase to hear in science, the one that heralds new discoveries, is not 'Eureka!' (I found it!) but rather, 'Hmmm... That's funny...'"
~Isaac Asimov

CHAPTER ONE

Myriam – a friend having similar difficulties – called in the afternoon.

"The pain feels like fire," she said. "It tingles and goes from the leg to inside my foot."

"I am going to see my new doctor tomorrow," she continued. "He is Dr. Rind. He is Chasid. He trained in acupuncture in China. Now, he has a private practice in White Flint. I went to him already once before. When he examines you, he doesn't touch you. He just moves his hand over your body. Then, he says, 'Your problem isn't in your back, it's in your hip', and he does something to move the hip into place. He doesn't charge, because my daughter-in-law is his cousin. Maybe you would like to go with me and meet him?..."

I called home.

"Things are okay," my brother said. "On Sunday I went surfing. It was kind of good to get my mind off law school. I guess that I feel about surfing is kind of like the same way that you treat dance."

Then, he checked himself.

"Mom's doing better," he continued. "The Psychiatrist put her on a new medication. She seems more up..."

The phone rang. It was Zev, the director of the Israeli dance troupe.

"How is your leg, Mike?" he asked. "We have plans to dance at George Mason University this weekend. You want to join us?... The group misses you. Are you getting better? How is that chiropractor that you went to? Are you still seeing him?... No?... Well, give this weekend some thought. If you can join us, the group would love to have you..."

1

Alone in bed, I turned out the light…

CHAPTER TWO

At the parking lot of the White Flint Mall, I waited for Myriam.

"Mike, come this way," she said. "I go through Lord & Taylor to get to Dr. Rind's clinic."

Through the basement we entered the loading elevator at the department store.

"You will like this doctor," she said. "He is very interesting."

At the women's section we made a turn at the blouses rack, that took us into the mall. After the Barnes and Noble we passed a secluded area called the Georgetown section, that contained a number of offices that appeared like small boutiques.

"Here is Dr. Rind's clinic," Myriam said.

A sign outside the door read The Health Institute.

"Hmm," I thought. "Impressive name for a tiny clinic."

We were escorted to an exam room that was gently lit.

"Why you haven't come over?" Myriam asked. "It's been a long time. I am cooking lamb this Friday. You come over then? I told the story about your mother to a friend... The one about how you told your mother about how you discovered the delicious marrow inside the lamb bone at my house, and she said she'd known all along, but wanted to save it for herself. All around the table everybody laugh..."

Then, a surge of electricity seemed to fill the air as a very ordinary looking, overweight man with intense beady-eyes entered the room.

"Okay, what's up?" he demanded. "What happened this time?"

Myriam responded with round-about answers.

"Well, I don't know," she said. "I hurt my back again... Mostly, it happens when I twist... Some of the time... Not all of the time..."

Then, he turned on me.

"What's your problem?" he asked.

I straightened, intent on keeping my responses to the point.

"I hurt my leg," I said.

He passed his hand behind me without touching me.

"You have something," he said. "But I haven't got time to work on you now. If you want to come back, you can make an appointment."

Then, without the slightest inhibition, he went about correcting the misalignments in Myriam's spine. I'd seen displays of medical prowess before, but none rivaled this. I felt like I was in the presence of a Master. He seemed like a mechanic of the body. Not only did he probe the body for subtle irregularities, he repaired them. Watching him, I felt awed and intimidated at the same time.

"Maybe I could learn from him?" I thought. "Maybe he'd teach me?..."

CHAPTER THREE

I scheduled an appointment with Dr. Rind. Arriving at the clinic I took a seat in the waiting area, and hunkered over my chair, anxiously recalled Dr. Rind's questioning of Miriam and wondered how I'd hold up to that?

Then, looking up, I saw a young woman staring back at me with kind, sympathetic eyes.

"Are you nervous?" she inquired. "Because it looks like if your shoulders were drawn up any closer, they'd be touching each other."

I smiled and relaxed my shoulders.

"I'm Elizabeth," she said. "My friends call me, Liz. I'm a patient of Dr. Weber's… He's the dentist here – He takes care of my TMJ [temporomandibular joint pain]."

Nodding, I noted the restricted movement of her jaw (like it was an effort to speak) and admired that it didn't keep her from smiling and carrying on in good humor.

"Mike," I responded. "I'm here to see Dr. Rind."

"I started seeing Dr. Rind, too," she responded. "Because I have abdominal problems. Dr. Rind thinks I have pancreatitis. He says it's probably because of gall stones. I hope he's right. I've been to all kinds of specialists and none of them have been able to help."

"I'm seeing him for a leg problem," I responded. "None of the specialists I've worked with were able to help me, either. And *I* wound up with abdominal problems because of all the nonsteroidal anti-inflammatory drugs they gave me caused an ulcer. In fact, it wasn't until a visiting scientist did acupuncture on me that I got better."

"I'm looking for an acupuncturist," she said. "Does he take patients?"

"No, he isn't here anymore," I replied. "He went back to Japan."
I sat, reflecting.

"It was amazing," I said. "He put those needles in and told me, 'Three days and the problem will be better.' I thought, 'No way. I've had this problem for months. It isn't gonna get better in no three days.' But, sure enough, three days later and the pain was gone."

"Wow," she said.

"Yeah, he had a reputation for being really good that way," I continued. "He'd been a post-doc in the lab I work at, and was known all over the NIH [National Institutes of Health] for helping scientists there. So when he returned for a visit, my boss insisted he work on me."

Then, as I remembered Hidemi told me that he had trained in acupuncture in China, it occurred to me that I had book on Chinese Medicine in my backpack.

"It talks about internal organ problems and offers suggestions for diet and pressure points to help," I said, digging through my pack. "I'll give it to you."

"Oh, I wouldn't want you to do that," she objected.

"It's no problem," I said. "I think you need it. I'll put my name and number in it, in case you'd like to get together and talk some more."

Handing her the text, she looked at me, surprised.

"That's funny," she said. "It felt like an energy passed through your book into my hand…"

A medical assistant appeared and called me back.

"I'm Renee," she said, escorting me to an exam room. "I'm Dr. Rind's medical assistant. He'll be with you in a minute…"

Although kind and attentive, she appeared pressed for time, and I wondered how backed up they were and how long I'd be waiting?

But in just a short time, there was a polite knock at the door, as it gently gave way.

"Oh, hi," said Dr. Rind. "How's it going?"

He was nothing like the man I'd met the other day; instead of intense and assertive, he was relaxed and easy-going.

"I don't think you have anything serious," he commented. "Probably a trigger point in your hamstring. It should clear up with an injection…"

After, he escorted me to the front desk.

"Dr. Rind, I'm a medical student," I said. "I'm currently doing research at the NIH, but I'm interested the work you're doing here. Is there any possibility I could volunteer?"

"Sure," he responded. "Come by whenever you want…"

CHAPTER FOUR

The next day I returned to the clinic.

"Oh!" Dr. Rind said, surprised. "You're back!"

He showed me to his personal library. It was crammed with books and papers.

"The work that I do here," he began, "follows from the teachings of Dr. Andrew Taylor Still. He was the founder of Osteopathy. Before that, he was a conventional doc who lived around the time of the Civil War. When he lost his family to disease and famine, he decided there had to be a better way to treat patients. So, he performed a detailed study of the human anatomy and came up with the holistic concept of the body as an integrated unit. Before that, Medicine followed the usual reductionist perspective of treating the body like a lot of disconnected parts. Instead of, 'Oh, it's the leg,' or 'It's your shoulder,' Dr. Still took the approach that an injury at one location could affect the body as a whole."

I nodded. These concepts were familiar to me, as my leg injury had led me to study practices like the Alexander Technique, Feldenkrais Method and others that talked about facilitating optimal motion and function through posture, alignment and proper use of the body.

"Then, he devised the concept of the key lesion," Rind continued. "It represents the actual site of injury - what lay behind all the superfluous layers of pain and symptoms. Just because a patient comes in with a sore neck doesn't mean that the problem has to be in his neck. It could be in the neck, but it could also be in the back or the foot.

"Say the guy has a problem with his foot, so he stands a little different. As a result, the back gets tilted. Then, to hold his head up

7

straight, he tilts his neck a certain way, and - Boom! - you have neck pain. The key lesion is in the foot. That's where the problem is. You have to treat the foot."

This is interesting, I thought. But how do you find this 'key lesion'? What points you to it?

"You see what I'm saying?" he inquired. "So far so good?... Are you with me?... Okay, I got to get rolling here. Let's start seeing patients."

Trailing behind him to the exam rooms, he signaled me to wait, then gently knocked on one of the doors and peeked inside.

"I have a young doctor," he whispered. "Would you mind if he came in and observed?"

He signaled me to follow. The patient was a young woman. She had dark hair and wore a joyless expression. He asked her some questions, then gently assisted her to a reclining position on the examining table. Without an explanation, he ran his hand over her abdomen without touching her, then called me over.

"Feel this," he said.

Stepping forward, I passed my hand over the patient's abdomen the way he had.

"Do you feel that?" he asked.

Oddly enough, I did feel something. It felt like a breeze blowing from her abdomen against my hand.

"What direction is it going?" Rind asked, matter-of-factly.

"Wait a minute," I insisted. "What is this?"

"Bioenergy," he muttered under his breath.

"What's that?"

"It's the body's way of pinpointing a blockage," he said. "Energy gets stuck at the site of injury; it can't move, so it just collects there. Now feel for what direction it's going."

"How do I do that?"

"Let the energy move your hand to whichever direction it wants to go," he instructed.

It moved my hand diagonally across her torso.

"That's right," he responded. "It's a stretch injury... Her body got wrenched against a seatbelt strap in an automobile accident. Now it needs to be corrected."

He removed a device from the drawer of a cabinet.

"This is a percussion hammer," he indicated. "It delivers a vibration that relaxes the muscles."

Applying the device to her abdomen, he gently guided it across until the muscles relaxed.

Leaving the examination room I walked into the hallway, stunned and speechless. Dr. Rind stood across from me. To my inquiring gaze, he just shrugged his shoulders – as though what he'd just shown me was nothing out of the ordinary...

CHAPTER FIVE

The hours and days that followed were the most exciting of my life! Moving from exam room to exam room, I watched Dr. Rind performed nothing less than medical miracles. There was no condition to complex for his mind to fathom, as he remedied ailments that his patients had been suffering for years – And treating all this as though it were commonplace?!

"Rule number one," Rind began. "Structure and function are related. If you understood the form well enough, you'll be able to understand the function. If you know the function, then you should be able to understand what the form should be. So, there's a relationship between them. It's extremely important in treating joints, for example…"

In my years in medical school and the NIH, I had trained with the acknowledged great practitioners of Medicine and beheld them demonstrate amazing feats of intellect when it came to an understanding of the intricacies of the body and disease; but none rivaled the kind of prowess that Dr. Rind displayed – Not only was he diagnosing these incredibly complex conditions, but he was healing them, too – And all this within the span of an office visit!

"In every joint there is an articulating surface, which is covered by smooth cartilage, and stabilizing structures called ligaments. In the ligaments there are fibers, like the cables supporting a bridge. They will only allow movement in certain directions, but disallow motion in other directions…"

Central to all of this was this phenomenon of Bioenergy – this mysterious energy emission that held the key to understanding what the patient needs.

"If you were to take a look at the bones of the skull, you would see that they have an articulating surface and are not fused. So, if you look at the form, you have to conclude that they move, and have the ability to permit cranial motion, and it's a pumping mechanism..."

To my unending surprise and disbelief, I found I could perceive it with every patient. And with each, Dr. Rind explained how it was that that energy was providing him with the roadmap for how to heal them.

And it was stunning, too, because at times this invisible force spoke so loudly!

An elderly woman brought in by family who said she suffered from nagging back pain. The woman looked ancient – so old and debilitated that she could barely speak.

What energy could she have? I thought. I couldn't imagine much.

Yet when I passed my hand behind her to scan her energetically, I felt what amounted to gale force winds blowing from her back!

Astonished, I stepped back.

This elderly woman?! I thought. Who could hardly communicate her needs?! How could this be?!

"But the regular doc says, 'They don't move.' You say, 'Why?', and he says, 'Because I can't feel them move.' It's the same with the sacro-iliac joint. The orthopedist will look at the ileo-sacral joint, and say, 'Oh, that's an immobile joint.' I say, 'Look, they have an articulating surface. They have shiny, smooth cartilage. They have ligaments - the strongest, most complex ligaments in the body - and you're telling me it doesn't move?' 'Yeah, it doesn't move,' they say, 'because I've never seen it move.'

"Then, I say to them, 'Well, what happens when take a mobile joint like a shoulder and immobilize it in a cast for six months?' What happens is, it becomes frozen - It just becomes one big piece of calcium, because it closes its articulating surface, it closes its ligaments, it closes everything, and becomes one big piece of bone. Because if it's not articulating, and it has no motion, the body gets rid of it. The body invests an amazing amount of energy to maintain the joints. If it doesn't need them, and isn't using them, it gets rid of them.

"Yet, orthopedic doctors will tell you, 'Those bones don't move.' They won't get it, because they won't recognize the simple principle that form and function are related."

"Okay, you got it now?" he asked. "That's number one. Next, the body has the inherent capacity to heal itself," he said. "It has intelligence and an innate ability for self-repair. Very little has to be said about that. That's the level that I do Bioenergy, and relates directly to that."

"Well, if the body is so capable of self-healing," I inquired, "why doesn't it just get better by itself?"

"It can," he responded. "It's just like you jumping from here to there. You can do it. But if I give you a little push, you'll start right away. We're just here to provide that little push."

But what was the source of this energy that he was teaching me. Was it physical? Spiritual? It appeared simple, as though anyone could do it, and yet I've never heard anything about it before.

"Now, if you talk to a regular MD," he continued, "he'll say, 'First of all, it's impossible, and, second, it can't be done.' Or, perhaps, he'd say, 'Okay, I believe that something's happened, but it's so rare that it's either bizarre or it's miraculous because you can't have such a profound effect with such a minor maneuver.' I do this all day, every day. It's become the stuff that I do. And it's the kind of stuff that I think every doctor should be able to do. But they're too busy poo-pooing this. You'd think that if somebody could do 'miracles,' they'd be asking how these techniques work, instead of telling patients that it's a load of crap, and 'It's witchcraft,' and 'The stuff doesn't work.' Their patients are like, 'Okay, if you say so. But what can I do? This other doctor is getting me better.'

"But what happens when I talk about these things, is I almost put myself out as a target. The medical community can point at me and say, 'Ah, you can't really believe in this stuff.' To them, if it isn't in the mainstream medical literature, it doesn't exist – the knowledge doesn't have any meaning to them. You wind up putting yourself at risk because doing this stuff doesn't correspond to what to them is 'normal' medicine…"

Near the end of the day, Dr. Rind complained of pain in his shoulder.

"Check the motion in the joint," he told me.

Stepping forward, I examined his range of motion.

"Oww!" he called out, good-naturedly.

But I'd barely lifted his arm, and having spent the day watching him perform what to me were nothing less than miracles, I couldn't imagine anything wrong with him. After all, he could fix anything – He'd been doing that for others all day. How could there possibly be anything wrong with him? As such, I'd expected him to have all the attributes of a yogi. But the motion in his shoulder was far worse and more restricted than any of the patients I'd examined that day.

Stunned, I stepped back.

"I'm sorry," I stammered. "I just thought… With everything you've taught me… I didn't think…"

He held his shoulder.

"I'm full of lesions!" he responded, still smiling.

Lowering my head, I expected to be severely reprimanded for my incorrect assumption, as I would have with any of my previous medical school attendings; instead, he patiently instructed me in an 'energy technique' for promoting the physical unwinding of locked joints.

"Put your hands on my shoulders," he said. "Now, I'm going to let go and you just follow where my body takes me."

He closed his eyes and oscillated back and forth as I secured him at the shoulders. Then, opening his eyes again, he swung his arm around, having seemingly recovered full range of motion in the shoulder.

"It's better," he said. "Thanks…"

CHAPTER SIX

At the newly opened Office of Alternative Medicine at the National Institutes of Health, I'd made arrangements to meet with the Deputy Director.

"I am Dr. Daniel Eskinazi," he said.

He spoke with a formal French accent. We shook hands and he led me to his office.

"Sit down," he said. "If I'm not mistaken, you work here, correct?"

"That's right," I said. "I'm a Howard Hughes scholar studying cancer vaccines at the National Cancer Institute."

"At what stage is your research?" he said.

"The FDA has cleared it for clinical trials," I said. "We've begun testing it in patients with advanced cancer."

"Very good," he said. "What brings you here?"

"About a year ago I injured my leg," I said. "I didn't get better with conventional modes of treatment, and, finally, resorted to alternative techniques. I've seen acupuncturists, chiropractors, and massage therapists. All have helped, and now I've found something that particularly sparks my interest."

"And what area of alternative medicine would that be?" he said.

"It's something called Bioenergy," I said. "It enables you to perceive energy imbalances, and locate abnormalities in the body that would otherwise go un-detect. It appears to be useful in determining the root cause of illness."

"Who has been showing you this technique?" he said.

"A physician named Dr. Bruce Rind," I said. "The experience of volunteering in his clinic has led me to re-evaluate my goals in medicine. Right now, I'm slated to return to medical school after I

14

complete my cancer vaccine project, but I want to pursue this new calling..."

"First," he interrupted, "I think that you should finish medical school. Only then can you act as a physician when applying what you've learned in alternative medicine, especially if you will be active in applying these techniques at the NIH. Practitioners of alternative medicine - osteopaths, chiropractors, acupuncturists - need to form their own lobby to facilitate national change. Research can be directed as a number of case studies, but collective groups of alternative therapy practitioners need to be assembled so that it can be done on a broader stage."

"I would like to meet this new doctor that you spoke of," he continued. "Yes, Dr. Rind. Do you think that he would come and see me?"

"I'll ask," I said.

"One last thing that I'm interested in," he said. "How did you injure your leg?"

I hesitated.

"I suppose that it's kind of complicated," I said. "I'd been dancing a lot, and I think that I put an undue amount of stress on the leg. Then, I went to New York to visit my uncle. While I was there, we were playing basketball, and the back of my leg began to cramp. My uncle saw some of our teammates working on similar sore muscles - the one with the leg problem would lie flat with his affect leg raised, while another applied pressure. My uncle tried this on me. But when he did, I felt something tear and snap. Afterwards, it just got worse."

He nodded.

"These kinds of injuries can be difficult to heal," he said.

"It certainly has led me to an interesting place," I responded.

He smiled and walked me to the door.

"I'll look forward to seeing you again," he said. "The next time I hope it will be with Dr. Rind..."

CHAPTER SEVEN

At the clinic Dr. Rind introduced me to a woman with bright smiling eyes and chipper, curt way of speaking.

"I have numbness between my fingers," she complained. "They ache."

"Gina is a flutist," Dr. Rind commented, "so problems like these pose an occupational hazard."

Chatting with Dr. Rind, Gina had a chipper, curt way of talking, with a tendency to gush and laugh as she spoke, even at dark humor. It all sang of a long forgotten melody of the beautiful sounds I left to pursue research in cancer vaccine development – They were the sounds of first love, Bubbles.

"Gina followed me from when I used to work at Reichstag Managed Care," Dr. Rind confided. "I worked there for a couple of years – That's where I got interested in pain management... I'm an anesthesiologist by training. I'd been overseeing one surgery after another for patients going under for so- called 'nerve impingement syndrome.' The usual routine is to make an incision near the area where the patient's having symptoms, then cut away the cartilage and chip at the bone. Theoretically, this is supposed to remove the source of impingement on the nerve. But, on follow up, I was finding that the patients had more problems after the procedure than they did before they came to the hospital."

Primum non nocere, I thought, nodding. First do no harm.

"This sort of thing enraged me," Rind continued. "Not only had the doctor not properly treated the problem, he'd actually done harm - And still charged the guy!

"I began spending more of my time in the pain clinic. In the evenings I attended continuing education classes in pain

16

management the way other people go out to dinner. I enrolled in course after course - acupuncture, osteopathy, cranial sacral therapy - and got certified in all of them.

"Then, I began asking the surgeons questions. I'd look over their shoulders during surgery, and say, 'Okay, guys, you've made the incision, now where's the impingement?' 'Oh, can't really see anything,' they'd say, 'but we'll just chip away at this area a little bit, anyway.'"

"When it got back to Administration, I was canned," he concluded...

Dr. Rind asked Gina to lay back on the table and then examined her back.

"She has a rotation between her second and third lumbar vertebrae," he said. "Feel it."

Palpating her vertebrae, I noted the bones felt out of alignment.

"Now, see what you feel when you scan her for energy disturbances," he said.

Moving my hand over her back, I perceived the sensation of a breeze between her shoulders.

"The energy is interesting," I said. "Over the right shoulder it's as though the energy is directing my hand inwards, whereas on the left, it's pushing my hand back."

"The fascial pulls are tugging her into the position of her vocation," he explained. "Holding a flute."

"Gina overdid it last summer," he continued. "She took too many jobs at outdoor events. Working days and evenings, and overstressed the muscles."

Just then, the muscles in her shoulder spontaneously jumped, so to signal a significant release, and when I looked for the energetic strain again, I couldn't find it.

"Look at her back," Dr. Rind instructed.

The vertebrae had lost their prior prominence and no longer felt out of alignment.

"It's as though everything went back into place," I said. "How did that happen?"

"A person who's been injured taps into your body to get relief," he said.

"What?!" I exclaimed. "How does my body know how to heal hers?"

"I don't know that it does know," he responded. "The body just does it..."

CHAPTER EIGHT

As the problems with my leg improved, I began performing with the Israeli dance troupe again.

After rehearsals, our director, Zev, pulled me aside.

"I've been telling my niece, April, about you," he said. "She's doing an internship at the Smithsonian. She wants to meet you..."

On Friday evening I joined Zev and his family for Shabbat. At the table I was seated next to April.

"I understand that you're a doctor," she said, "and had an injury that's changed the way you look at Medicine."

"I'm a medical student," I replied. "And, yes, the injury has led me to see things differently."

"What things?" she said.

"Medication," I responded, blithely. "Treatment. My doctors told me that I wouldn't walk normally again and could expect chronic pain for life. They gave me all kinds of medicines: NSAIDs, which caused an ulcer; muscle relaxants that made me feel like I was sleeping my life away. None of them helped – they just made the situation worse."

She listened intently.

"I have a friend who became an acupuncturist," she commented. "She also had a problem that wouldn't get better. She went to China to study Traditional Chinese Medicine. Now, she teaches it in this country. I've tried to talk to her about it, but she insists that it's necessary to experience illness before you can comprehend other forms of healing."

A sick feeling crept over me.

"Then, I hope you'll never understand," I said...

CHAPTER NINE

In the exam room the patient looked uncomfortable.

"Mr. Blevins came to the clinic looking for relief of his shoulder pain," Dr. Rind explained. "Why don't you examine him?"

Scanning him energetically, I found energy radiated from his shoulders, and there were taut bands of muscle stretched across the trapezius muscles on both sides.

"I've found the trigger points," I said.

Dr. Rind smiled.

"Watch this," he said.

He pressed the patient's palms. To my amazement, the energy dissipated, and the muscles over his shoulder - which had been as tight as guitar strings - melted under my fingertips. Then, Dr. Rind took his hand away, and the taut bands returned. I looked at him, stunned.

"How did you do that?" I asked.

"Look at Mr. Blevins' hands," he said.

The patient's palms were so scarred they could barely open.

"It happened when I was an infant," Mr. Blevins said. "My mother said that I was crawling around when I put my hands on the radiator."

"The scars in his hands are still sending pain signals to the body," Dr. Rind said. "In return, the body overcompensates by creating contractions at the shoulders."

"So, the scars are the key lesion," I said. "But how were you able to get rid of the taut bands in his shoulders by just pressing his palms?"

"By focusing my intention there," he answered. "When you provide another sensory stimulus, you nullify the painful one."

"How does that happen?" I asked.

"By finding the correct site of injury," he said. "When you identify the problem, the body stops sending a pain message. It's like the body breathes a sigh of relief. 'Ahh,' it says, 'he's finally found the problem.'"

"But how would I find it, if I didn't see the scars?" I asked.

"Energetically," he said. "With your one hand, feel for the energy at the patient's shoulders. Then, when you've done that, with your other hand, scan the patient's palms."

As soon as I became aware of the perception of energy at the patient's palms, the energy at the shoulders disappeared.

"By finding the correct site of injury," Rind explained, "you identify the primary problem. As soon as that happens, the body stops sending the pain message, and the energy imbalances elsewhere become neutralized."

Dr. Rind prepared a mixture and injected the scars. Soon the contractures in the palms softened, and the muscle spasms in the patient's shoulders had disappeared.

"The Chinese have a saying," Rind said. "'You can treat the leaves or you can treat the roots.' In other words, you can stay up all night painting the leaves green, or you could simply give the plant some water. It's the same way in Medicine."

The patient swung his arms around.

"They feel a lot better," Mr. Blevins said...

CHAPTER TEN

A pleasant young woman came to the clinic for the first time.

"I was rear-ended several months back," she said. "Since then, I've been having problems with my neck."

With the patient's permission, Dr. Rind invited me to examine her.

"Follow the tension in the fascial planes," Rind instructed. "As you examine her, provide gentle support."

But even as I supported her neck, it was as though it wanted to arch so far back that I feared it would separate from her head.

Nevertheless, the patient didn't indicate the least discomfort; indeed, it seemed to provide a sense of ease to her.

"Why is it doing this?" I asked.

"Her body is re-living the accident," Rind responded. "At the time her head was forced all the way back. The body has a memory of the trauma. It's your job to tap into that."

Her neck extended even further.

"I'm afraid she's going to hurt herself," I said.

"Focus on the structures of the cervical vertebrae," he instructed.

Creating a mental image of her neck bones, the patient's head began to straighten.

"It's better," I said. "But I noticed that when her neck went back, it seems to be arcing to one side."

"That's important," he said. "Then, it's probably not a midline structure, like the bones. The X-rays didn't show any evidence of fracture. More likely, it's a muscular injury."

"How do we find it?" I asked.

"You rely on the fascial planes to get a feeling for what happened during the time of injury," he said.

Following the fascial planes, her neck assumed a position all the way back and to the side. Then, all at once, her body began to bounce as though on a roller coaster ride.

"What's happening?" I asked.

"When you arrive at the position of injury, her body re-lives the accident," he said.

"That little bump could do all this?!" the patient said.

"Yep," Rind responded.

He turned back to me.

"In her movements are all the events that happened during the collision," he said. "The body is replaying an exact recreation of those events. You can see the whole accident in the movements that she's making. The body is trying to come to terms with an event that caught her off guard."

"Now it's begging for assistance," I thought.

"The body knows what it needs," Rind said. "It's there waiting to tell you. It's just a matter of knowing how to listen..."

CHAPTER ELEVEN

Returning to the Office of Alternative Medicine with Dr. Rind, I introduced him to Dr. Eskinazi.

"Mike told me a little about the work you do," Dr. Eskinazi said. "What kind of cases do you usually see in your clinic?"

Dr. Rind shrugged.

"I don't know," Rind responded, nonchalantly. "I can tell you about the cases that I saw today. I had a follow-up visit from a 14 year old girl. She'd been having headaches. She'd already undergone four craniotomies for benign tumors, and was about to have another. I localized the source of headaches to a trigger point in her right shoulder. With a little massage, the headaches went away. The patient's father says to me that the MRIs had cost $5,000; the previous surgeries, another $25,000. What you did was easily worth a million!'"

Dr. Eskinazi leaned back in his chair, spellbound and smiling as though almost unable to contain himself, as Dr. Rind described case after case.

"I have two girls right now who are patients of mine," Dr. Rind continued. "One is 25, the other is 35. Both were blind when they came to me. One was blind for about 2 or 3 years. The other was blind for 10 years. I'm talking about legally blind, with the dark glasses and the stick and the whole business. One I treated with IV therapy and it got the patient back to the point where she's able to read and use the computer.

"The other one - who was a type 1 diabetic - I said, 'We have to change your diet because your body is having difficulty breaking foods down,' and I put on some very serious nutrients and antioxidants and gave her IV therapy to energize her body, and she started to see a lot better and her body started to be able to heal.

"At that point she was able to undergo a surgery, which before that she was unable to do. But now her surgeon said, 'You're healthy enough and strong enough to be able to do it.' And she did. Now, she has 20/40 vision. She can drive without glasses. She was legally blind for ten years."

"Now, with these two girls," he concluded, "the average doc would say, 'These are miracles.' And I'm telling you right now, these are not miracles - They're simply an application of basic principles..."

Leaving the building, Rind pulled me aside.

"On the one hand, I wanted to score as many points as I could with this guy," he said. "But, on the other, I didn't want to underscore your contribution."

I shook my head.

"I don't feel slighted," I said. "I just want this stuff to come out, so that patients can benefit."

Dr. Rind looked away.

"I'm barely able to make a living," he confided. "I just work in my office and don't have the time to go out and try to get things happening. Maybe, you do. Maybe, you can get some of these things to grow. There's just so much that I can do."

"Perhaps, you can write a book?" I said.

"There are plenty of osteopathic texts out there," he responded.

"I've never seen any that describe your techniques," I said.

"Who'd publish it?" he queried.

"Maybe the same people who've published the books you've lent me?" I said.

"I'll give it some thought," he replied. "But if you're going to be a co-author, I want you to have your MD. I don't want you to be a poor student anymore. It doesn't open as many doors..."

CHAPTER TWELVE

"There's another way to perceive what's going on in a patient," Dr. Rind told me.

We were in an exam room with his patient, Mr. Penn. Dr. Rind instructed the patient to lie with his back against the examining table.

"Mike, stand at the foot of the table and grip the patient's ankles," Dr. Rind said. "Now, try to open yourself to any new sensations."

All at once I experienced a fatigue and heaviness along my chest and abdomen. Then, a pain in my lower back developed. It was sharp pain, mostly on the right. I tried to get past it, but it seemed that I was stuck there, and my muscles were clamping down. I looked at Dr. Rind.

"What is this?" I asked.

"Interlink," Dr. Rind said. "It's a means of energy transfer… The body is crying out for a connection. It wants to tell you what it needs."

I clamped my eyes shut and tried to tolerate the feeling.

"Mr. Penn, where is the majority of your pain?" I asked.

"In my back," he responded.

"Which side?"

"On the right."

I hung on, but the discomfort was intense.

"Dr. Rind, I can't seem to get beyond the feeling that I'm getting from his back," I said. "I seem to be stuck - I can't move any lower. Is there anything that I can do?"

"Let go of his ankles," he responded.

I took my hands away; within an instant, the intense tightness encircling my lower back was gone. I looked about, startled.

"That's it?" I asked. "It's that simple?"

"That's it," Rind responded, casually. "The body's said what it needed to tell you."

"No?!" I thought.

I clasped the patient's ankles again - the fatigue and heaviness in my chest reappeared, then the clamping sensation in my back. I let go - it evaporated. I looked to Dr. Rind.

"It can't be?"

I tried a third time - the same result.

"Now, let's correct it," Rind declared.

Dr. Rind instructed the patient turned over on the table. Examining his back, I found there were thick bands of muscle, stretching midline from his spine all the way to his sides.

"What is this?" I asked.

"Muscle irritation," Rind responded. "It represents disorderly muscular contractions."

"So, do these disorderly contractions ever cut off the blood supply to the muscle and cause them to die?"

"No," he responded. "When the contraction cuts off too much blood, lactic acid builds up – As a result the vessel vasodilates and feeds the muscles a little bit. After that, the whole process starts all over again."

Rind applied gentle percussion.

"What does that do?" I asked.

"It reduces the congestion in the area."

As he worked on the patient's back I felt a sensation of energy in my hands. I rubbed them against my sides, but the feeling wouldn't go away.

"Mr. Penn, are you feeling anything?" I said.

"I'm experiencing a tingling in my hands," he said.

I looked at Dr. Rind.

"How can this be?" I thought.

Examining the patient, the thick bands of muscle were supple now.

Getting up from the table, Mr. Penn smiled broadly.

"Thanks," he said. "This is the best that I've felt in a good long while..."

CHAPTER THIRTEEN

A well-off Romanian man sat impatiently in the examining room.

"I have this chest pain," he said. "It won't go away. I've been to the best specialists. I just came from the Mayo Clinic. None of them could tell me what to do about it."

Dr. Rind scanned him, then asked me to do the same.

"There's a focus of energy radiating from his chest," I said.

"Where in the chest?" Rind asked. "How deep is it?"

"I don't know," I responded. "How would I figure that out?"

"Envision a ruler, then count through the inches," he said. "When you get to the right level, you'll feel the energy give out."

"Why does it do that?"

"Because you've temporarily reconciled the body with the source of injury by focusing your energy there," he said. "Pain is there to tell you something. It's the body's way of saying 'It's right here. Now do something about it.' When you address the wound, the body responds by saying 'Oh, he's got the message' and turns down the volume."

I conceived a ruler: At three inches the energy faded.

"What kind of tissue is involved?" he asked.

"I don't know," I said. "How do I determine that?"

"Picture in your mind what muscle looks like and what lung is," he said. "Then, see what the energy feels like."

I envisioned the different tissues of the body: Forming an image of the lung (with its intricate webs of life-giving tissue), the energy radiating from the patient's chest diminished.

"Now, what is the process?" Rind persisted.

"What do you mean, 'process'?" I asked.

"Is it inflammation?" he said. "Is it a scar? Is it a granuloma? Is it an infection? Visualize in your mind what each of these looks like."

Drawing from my knowledge and experience in Pathology, I recalled and envisioned a number of microscopic images. The first involved immune cells attacking an infection. When this begot no response from the energy that emanated from the patient, I changed the image to one in which those cells were dying, leaving calcified remnants in their wake. Still, no response. Finally, I conjured an image of a trail of fibrotic tissue. In that moment, the energy diminished.

"It's a scar," I said.

"Did you have any bad lung infections when you were younger?" Rind asked the patient.

"I had tuberculosis in secondary school," the patient responded. "I told this to my other doctors, but nothing had ever shown up on chest X-ray or CT scan, so they dismissed it."

Dr. Rind turned to me.

"You see," he said, "the scars from these infections are often so subtle they can't be seen on imaging studies. Nevertheless, they create significant tugs on the fascial planes of the body, provoking misalignments and pain."

Dr. Rind instructed the patient in breathing exercises to treat the scarring. Standing in a corner of the room, my thoughts were clouded with awe and amazement, as I considered the possibilities.

Innate abilities to diagnose and localize disease? I thought. Invisible signals from the body to attune to?

"There's great value in looking at things with these other perspectives," Rind asserted, "and taking whatever skills you have and applying some good wholesome principles to those areas. We have skills that we never really apply."

"These are very simple principles which, on the surface, seem ridiculously simple at first glance," he continued. "But, then, you realize that when doctors ignore these basic principles, they do very foolish things, and they miss the mark almost every time..."

CHAPTER FOURTEEN

In Taos, New Mexico at the Keystone Symposia, scientists gathered around my cancer vaccine poster.

"So you got it to work in the test tube?" they asked. "Good... How long will it be before you start clinical trials?... Has it been FDA-approved?... Congratulations..."

In the afternoon, most of my colleagues went skiing. I toured the ancient Native American pueblo, looked out at the cliff dwellings, then stared into the expansive clear blue sky.

"The cancer vaccine may one day save many lives," I thought. "But it won't stop the ravages of other diseases that will plague these patients."

The pueblo was closed off for the observation of a religious holiday, but walking past – even from miles away – it felt like I could perceive a chorus of chanting coming from the caves.

"Bioenergy it seems has the potential to help with so many things," I continued thinking.

After the conference, most of my colleagues were worn out from their days of skiing. As most slept during the long bus ride back to the airport in Santa Fe, I reached into my bag for a pen and paper.

"Bioenergy," I wrote. *"The Ultimate Diagnostic Tool..."*

CHAPTER FIFTEEN

Dr. Rind handed me back the treatise on Bioenergy I'd written.

"You read it?" I asked.

"Yeah," he said, distracted.

"What did you think?" I queried.

"It was okay," he responded.

He looked away from my inquiring glance.

"I tried to capture the essence of what you'd taught me," I said. "Is there something I left out?"

"Yeah," he said, distant.

I peered into his features. He hid his beady eyes.

"What?" I asked.

He shrugged.

"You can use it to heal..."

CHAPTER SIXTEEN

April accompanied Zev to rehearsals. Usually her hands weaved through the dance, but tonight something seemed different.

"I hurt my wrist," she said. "Is there anything that you've learned at the clinic that can help?"

A feeling of energy emanated from her forearm. Following its path, it led my hand outward. When the energy had completed its path, it felt as though the energy were squarely in my palm.

"How is the pain in your wrist, April?" I asked.

"It's gone," she said.

She moved her wrist around and there was a healthy snap. She looked up, startled.

"It feels like everything just went back into place," she said.

She smiled.

"So, you could feel something when you had your hand over my arm?" she asked.

"That's right," I said. "Energy radiated from your arm. It was the marker of an underlying injury. In turn, it can be used to facilitate healing."

"How do you heal using energy?" she asked.

"Follow it," I said. "Take the energy where it wants to go."

"Then what?"

"It balances the underlying energy strain."

"Why does it do that?" she asked.

"Because the body becomes reconciled with the source of trauma," I said. "Injury usually occurs because the muscle has been strained. Your body responds by tightening down. It says, 'I don't trust this person anymore - I'm never going to let him do that again.' So it stays contracted. The problem is, it takes the body out of

31

alignment and creates pain. It's detrimental to the body because, now, it's not able to perform its usual tasks. Bioenergy seeks to reconcile the body with the source of trauma - say to the body, 'Look, I know that you've been injured, but by staying like this, you're doing more harm than good.' The body hears this, and responds by letting go, and returning to its normal state. The body needs to be reconciled with the source of trauma before it can heal."

She looked away.

"My main area of study in college is Archaeology," she said, "but I'm also interested in Psychology. I've been studying what happens to little girls whose mothers are constantly beaten by their husbands... When the girls play with dolls, they represent the male doll beating the female repeatedly over the head. To them, this is perfectly natural. The trauma has drastically altered or even implanted a misperception of male-female relationships."

I sat back.

"Hmmm," I thought aloud. "Emotional scars?"

I looked at her.

"I wonder," I said. "Can Bioenergy be used to heal the traumas of childhood?..."

CHAPTER SEVENTEEN

After dancing I met Liz at a café.

"How was your rehearsal, Mike?" she asked.

"I had a good time," I said. "April and I danced. It was strange... When I dance with her, all the pain in my leg goes away. I don't know what that is?"

"It's euphoria," she responded. "That's the effect of euphoria. Loving someone has that effect. I think the whole basis for meditation in general is to be able to feel euphoria within. That's why it has a healing effect."

"Don't misunderstand me," she added. "The point of meditation is not so you don't need anybody else. It's not that at all. It makes you more approachable and loving towards others. It works both ways..."

CHAPTER EIGHTEEN

Dr. Rind pulled Renee and me aside to teach us Osteopathic maneuvers.

"There is no danger in a manipulation done right," he told us. "There is essentially no force needed. All it takes is a working knowledge of the anatomy. From there, the correct position can be easily ascertained. Put the body in the position it desires, and it will do the rest by itself. It just needs a little push to get it back into alignment, that's all."

"Renee, try it on Mike first," he said, "since he's a lot smaller than I am."

She had a delicate touch; a pop of my spine under her was like the snapping of the smallest of twigs.

"The better the position," Dr. Rind said, "the less force needed."

"I don't want to have to use any force at all," I thought.

"Now, Mike, you try it on me," he said.

With a minimum of force, I corrected misalignments in Dr. Rind's back.

"I feel so much better," he said. "Like I'm floating."

He lay smiling on the table. I was about to gently assist him off when a knock came from the door.

"Dr. Rind, you're 3 o'clock patient is here," said the secretary.

The next thing I knew, Dr. Rind's legs were near straight in the air! Falling with a loud crash, he bounced off the table.

"Back to work," he said...

CHAPTER NINETEEN

Accompanying Elizabeth to an appointment with Dr. Rind, we sat waiting in the exam room.

"Sorry I'm late," Dr. Rind said, entering the room. "I just came back from a seminar in holographic music."

"What's that?" I asked.

"It's music that's meant to activate the energy centers," he responded. "Let me demonstrate it for the two of you."

He arranged the treatment room, so that Elizabeth and I occupied separate examining tables on opposite sides of the room. Then, he played a tape of holographic music.

As the music played I envisioned black and yellow forms blending into one another – like images in a kaleidoscope – and sensed that Elizabeth was hovering over me. Opening my eyes, I expected to see her standing over me; instead, I found she was still on the other side of the room! And closing my eyes again, the blending black and yellow patterns returned...

"I had a vision," Elizabeth commented after the music finished. "It was a vision of contentment: Mike was smiling in a relaxed pose with his hand on his hip. Behind him, I saw a black and yellow design and had the feeling like somehow our bodies were coalescing together – as though we weren't composed of solid forms, but could freely flow into one another..."

CHAPTER TWENTY

Dr. Rind introduced me to a patient in an examination room.

"Mr. Helfman suffers from depression," Dr. Rind said. "His son is autistic. Usually, his source of strain is at the solar plexus. Examine him and see where it's coming from today."

Energy radiated from his shoulders.

"I didn't find anything at the solar plexus," I said. "Instead, I felt something from the shoulders."

"How do you interpret that?" Dr. Rind asked.

"If we're talking about emotional strains," I said, "from what I've been reading, problems at the shoulders could mean hold back feelings of anger."

Dr. Rind smiled, then looked at the patient.

"Yeah," Mr. Helfman affirmed. "I called Dr. Rind this afternoon saying I needed a treatment because I was feeling all of this pent up frustration."

"I've been having a hard time coping with my son's condition," he continued. "I keep asking, 'Why, God? Why?' I guess that I'm just mad at the world these days."

Dr. Rind treated him with acupuncture.

"What do you feel now, Mike?" Dr. Rind said.

Energy radiate outward from the patient's feet.

"What does it mean?" I asked.

The patient smiled.

"Well, I feel better," Mr. Helfman commented. "Maybe the bad energy   is   moving   out..."

CHAPTER TWENTY-ONE

At the National Institutes of Health a course was offered in Neural Networks.

"In this class," the professor began, "we will address the question, Can thoughts be mapped to defined regions? In particular, we'll pose the question, Can emotions be represented in the brain?"

On the blackboard, the professor drew a series of intricate diagrams detailing various cascading neural pathways.

In the meantime, my mind wandered.

"How could neural networks experimentally demonstrate the effective use of Bioenergy?" I thought.

"Programs have been designed," the professor said, "to test the hypothesis of how ideas are conducted in the brain."

Listening, I thought about patients at Dr. Rind's clinic.

Then, suddenly, I sat bolt upright in the chair.

"An EMPATH program," I thought. "I need to design an EMPATH program..."

CHAPTER TWENTY-TWO

"What we need to do," I told Dr. Rind, "is design and create a reliable means of tapping into the body and discovering what it needs to get well – Harnessing empathy to define medical treatment."

"We'd hook the patient up to a machine that could measure the energy coming off the body," I continued. "Like a full body EEG. An automated probe would then scan the body and locate the site of the primary lesion, just as performed in the neutralization technique. Focusing on the lesion, the EMPATH program could run through on infinite series of computer-generated diagnoses. In no time, a match could be generated – We'd simply wait for the energy in the body to become balanced and bring the body into alignment. It would be interlink between man and machine."

Dr. Rind appeared distracted.

"What do you think?" I inquired.

He shrugged his shoulders.

"Yeah, maybe," he said.

He looked away.

"Well, it's just information, right?" I said. "Interlink is just a matter of coming up with the correct diagnosis. Then, everything else falls into place. There isn't anything else to it is there?…"

CHAPTER TWENTY-THREE

"Let's play a game," Dr. Rind said, smiling.

I had been standing in the back of the exam room as Dr. Rind evaluated a middle-aged woman complaining of abdominal pain.

"I'm going to draw a picture of what I see is wrong with the patient," he said. "We'll compare it after we see what you find."

"Okay," I said.

Energy radiated from her eye.

"Is that the primary lesion?" Dr. Rind said.

Holding one hand over her eye, I scanned the rest of her body with my other hand.

"No," I said. "There's something coming from the lower part of her abdomen - on the right side."

"Is it the appendix or ovary?" he asked.

I visualized each.

"It's the ovary," I responded.

"What is the process?"

I visualized a number of ovarian conditions: Adhesions - the energy radiating from the ovary remained the same. Endometriosis - the energy persisted. Infection - no change.

Then, the image of an ovulatory cyst came to mind.

"Hmm?" I thought. "That's interesting. Wouldn't think that I'd come up with that one? – More like something that a specialist in Gynecology dreams up."

But scanning her now, the energy was gone.

I whipped my head around and looked at Dr. Rind.

"Cyst," I declared, startled. "Ovulatory cyst."

Dr. Rind smiled, then pulled out the paper and handed me the drawing he'd tucked away. I unfolded the paper – On it he'd drawn a well-demarcated dot within an oval – essentially a perfect representation of a cyst within an ovary!

"No?!" I exclaimed. "It can't be!..."

CHAPTER TWENTY-FOUR

Riding bikes with a fellow Howard Hughes scholar named Aaron, I confided my ambivalence for continuing conventional medicine training.

"I want to pursue natural healing," I said. "I've stumbled upon it, but now it's become something of a calling."

"I think it's the worst thing that you could do," he declared.

"Why?" I asked.

"Because they'll balk at you without pity."

"What could they do?" I inquired. "Would there be anything that I could tell them?"

But he just rode off in the other direction...

Awakening from the dream, I felt alone and uncertain...

CHAPTER TWENTY-FIVE

Dr. Rind returned from a conference in New York.

"I met Ethan Coleman," he said. "He's a renown healer from Israel. He showed us how to visualize auras."

"How do you do that?" I asked.

"It's like looking at the sun," he said. "When you close your eyes, you still see the image in the position that it was before. It's the same with the internal energy radiating from the body. It remains imprinted on the retina."

"Try it on me," he continued. "Look at me, then close your eyes and see what you still perceive on your retina."

Closing my eyes, shiny golden rods radiated from the position of his right shoulder.

"Now, scan me and see what you find," he said.

"There's a vector of energy radiating from your shoulder, alright," I said.

"I had a bad fall on it years ago," he responded. "I've had problems with it ever since..."

CHAPTER TWENTY-SIX

Zev pulled me aside during dance rehearsals.

"It looks like you are doing a lot better," he said. "That new doctor must be helping you. Maybe I should go and see him?... The problems in my back are acting up."

"He's taught me a lot of his techniques," I said. "If you like, maybe we can get together and I could try to help?"

"Alright," he said. "How about at my house tomorrow afternoon?..."

Before leaving for Zev's, I'd been reading an article in Dr. Rind's clinic about craniosacral therapy.

"Let me show you," I told Zev. "I'm going to cradle your head in my hands. The cranial rhythm is like a breathing cycle for the nervous system. It originates at the skull, and then traverses the entire body at a rate of eight to twelve cycles per minute. Where there's an uneven expansion of the cranium, it usually represents an unresolved trauma."

Following Zev's cranial rhythm, it felt locked on the right side.

Then, suddenly, I lost the rhythm; in its place was a minute vibration that felt like a trembling all around Zev's head.

"Mike, I'm feeling something," Zev said.

"What are you feeling?" I said.

"I don't know," he responded. "It's like a current streaming down my head."

"Are you okay?"

"Yes," he said. "It's a pleasurable feeling. But I feel like I can't open my eyes."

"Something like this happens to me at night sometimes," he continued. "If I force my eyes open, the feeling goes away, but usually returns when I go back to sleep again."

After a few minutes, the rhythm returned; however, now it was fuller than before, without the previous unevenness.

Zev rose and twisted from side to side.

"The pain in my back is gone," he declared. "I couldn't do that before without feeling it get caught on the right."

He smiled.

Still, I looked on, stunned.

What just happened? I thought...

CHAPTER TWENTY-SEVEN

"Still point!" Dr. Rind asserted, matter-of-factly.

I'd barely finished telling him about Zev.

"'Still point'?" I repeated. "What's that?"

"It's when the cranial rhythm stops, and repairs happen in all the places in the body where the cranial rhythm is weak," he said. "This is when most of the healing occurs. The rhythm comes back when the healing is complete."

"But there was nothing about still points in the pamphlet you gave me," I said.

"It's very advanced," he said. "The pamphlet was meant for beginners. Usually, beginners don't experience still points."

"What is the basis of cranial sacral therapy?" I said. "How does it work?"

"Trauma causes energy blockages," he responded. "Remember, the body is an integrated system, so its affects are registered everywhere, including the cranial rhythm. Cranial sacral therapy is another way of identifying the effects of trauma. When the cranial rhythm goes back to normal, it's usually because the energy blockage has been removed."

"You can actually perceive the cranial rhythm anywhere on the body," he continued. "It originates from the brain, but, from there, it follows the nerves and travels all over the body. You can feel it on me."

He laid on the examining table, and I felt for his cranial rhythm. It moved evenly over his head, but stopped over his shoulder.

"It's as though your right shoulder isn't breathing," I said. "What do I do now?"

"Let the patient's body taps into yours," he said. "It's like it's learning from you how to function normally again. It's forgotten because it's been traumatized. It's like a deer in the headlights. When we're caught off guard, we have a tendency to freeze. It's like that everywhere in the body.

"Afterwards, it has to relearn how to do things again. When you perform a technique like cranial sacral therapy, you connect with the patient's system. When a still point occurs, it's like the patient's body is saying, 'Oh, that's how it should be done,' and registers the correction."

"We've done something like this before, haven't we?" I said. "When you asked me to examine your shoulder shortly after I started here."

"That's right," he said. "I was tapping into your system."

"Like interlink," I thought.

As he spoke, the rhythm stopped. I looked at the clock. Within a minute the rhythm had resumed, only, now, it included his right shoulder.

"Thanks," he said. "My shoulder was bothering me again. It feels better now."

I nodded.

"It's all about interlink," I thought...

CHAPTER TWENTY-EIGHT

Elizabeth invited me to meet her mother, Lena, who was visiting from Rhode Island. My first impression was that she walked with an usual gait – wobbling from side to side.

"Mom, how long have you walked this way?" Elizabeth said.

"I couldn't say," she said. "For years... I don't have any pain. It's just difficult for me to walk straight."

"Mike, what do you think could have set it off?" Liz asked.

"I don't know," I said. "It could be a lot of things. Often, at the clinic, Dr. Rind treats patients with walking difficulties for surgical scars and pelvic trauma."

Lena thought.

"Maybe it was from having six children?" Lena said. "I also needed an appendectomy and cholecystectomy?"

"Mike, why don't you try doing Bioenergy on her," Liz said.

The energy that radiated from Lena seemed to fill the room.

"I've never experienced anything like this before," I said.

Following the energy's path took me across the room; it made its way through windows, and into walls, and, at times, I required a chair to reach high enough

In the meantime, Lena, who'd been sitting on the couch, had fallen asleep.

"She has narcolepsy," Liz said. "Should I wake her?"

"No, let her sleep," I said. "I'm feel embarrassed, anyways."

Lena awoke shortly after I'd finished.

"I'm sorry that I fell asleep," she said.

As she got up and walked across the room, Liz jumped back.

"Mom, you're walking straight," Liz called out.

"I am?" Lena said.

She walked back to the couch – Again, there wasn't a trace of her former wobble. Liz turned to me.

"Mike, that's amazing," she said...

CHAPTER TWENTY-NINE

The next day Lena and I accompanied Elizabeth to an appointment at the clinic.

"Hey guys," Dr. Rind said, cheerfully entering the exam room. "How are you doing?"

"Not so good," Liz responded. "The two sides of the brain didn't feel even."

"'Don't feel even?'" I thought. "What does that mean?"

He examined Elizabeth's reflexes.

"Her reflexes are all unequal," he said. "The right biceps is different from the left. The right knee is different. The right ankle is different from left ankle. It's that way all over the place."

Repeating his examination, I nodded.

"Yes, it's like it's dead on the right side, and hyper on the left," I said. "What could account for that?"

"Did you ever have a head injury?" Rind asked.

"She had a concussion when she was an infant," Lena said. "She was swinging on a rocking horse and fell off. She landed so hard that she lost consciousness. When I took her to the emergency room, the doctors insisted that she stay overnight for observation and testing. The next morning, though, they said that she was alright, and I took her home. She didn't appear then to have any problems, but I was always concerned there seemed to be something different."

"Well, I think that she had some kind of a central trauma," Rind responded, "because there's something going on way up in the brain. Let's check your cranial motion."

He cupped her head in his hands.

"Part of the temporal bone on the right side isn't moving well," he said. "What happened on this side?"

"That's where she fell," Lena said.

Dr. Rind looked at me.

"Okay, fine," he said. "So, confirmation. Look, I think the fall stunned the temporal joint. Next, at this point, we have to straighten out the temporal bone in the head, because essentially that's what's going on."

"How do you do that?" I asked.

"It's an osteopathic maneuver," he said. "It's about 5% manual and 95% Bioenergy."

He closed his eyes and focused.

Lena edged closer.

"Dr. Rind, I work at the school as a child psychologist," she said. "Have you ever treated children with learning disabilities?"

"Yeah, sure," he said. "I have one patient whose son is autistic. Mike, you remember Mr. Helfman?... Well, this is his autistic son. I gave the parents a few exercises to do with the child to improve the kid's cranial motion, and, after that, everything changed. His whole affect changed. Now, the son's improved so that he's got to a point where he's able to function with normal children now. This was an autistic kid. The same child who was incapable of tying his own shoe laces earlier. He's started to talk clearly, and wasn't staring out into space anymore.

"And he's doing very well. He's living like a balanced child. Mr. Helfman says that he's expanded his interests. He never had an interest in anything. He never wanted to try anything. Now, he trying new things. He's doing new things. He's running around. He's asking to learn new things. His mother home schools him. She says, 'He's asking me to teach him, and I'm having to keep up with him now, instead of the other way around.' And this was an autistic kid.

"In fact, they put him in summer camp. This is a kid that before that barely able to speak. Now, he's speaking, and getting along with everybody.

"This is what's interesting, though. At the beginning of the camp, they had a party for everybody. They're all sitting at a table, and one of the girls starts to choke. She starts to point at her throat, and everybody is sort of like staring at her, as she's turning blue. And this kid, with autism, walked over behind her, grabbed her under the rib cage, did a Heimlich maneuver. The pizza popped out across the table, and he went back to his chair, sat down, and continued eating his pizza. Everybody there was just shocked. The kid got a gold star for it."

Lena nodded.

"There is so much potential out there," she said. "Just think what could happen if other autistic children got the same treatment?"

Dr. Rind stood.

"Alright, we're done," he said. "Liz, you rest here on the examining table for a few minutes. Lena, please stay with her and let me know if anything happens... Mike, come with me, I have an interesting case I want to show you in the other room..."

Dr. Rind and I were still talking about the other patient when I noticed Lena standing in the hallway looking concerned.

"I think that you ought to see something," she said.

We followed her back to the room. Inside, Elizabeth looked out as though uncertain.

"What's going on, Liz?" I asked.

"I...," then, before she could produce a word more, her eyes spontaneously began darting back and forth in her head. The movement was too fast to be voluntary. It was as though the muscles behind her eyes were in a violent tug of war.

I stepped back and turned to Dr. Rind.

"What's happening?" I asked.

"Neuromuscular re-education," Dr. Rind responded, matter-of-factly. "The brain is reacquainting itself with the muscles of the body. The head injury that she had when she was young occurred at a time when her brain was still developing. The trauma shut down the development of more sophisticated pathways. It had to resort to the less sophisticated pathways that were already established. But these were pathways that should have been passed a long time ago, like early milestones in development. She's been relying on these old pathways all this time. Now, the sophisticated portions of the brain are reacquainting themselves with the body."

Elizabeth's eyes stopped moving. She breathed a sigh of relief.

"Whew," she said.

But, then, her body shuddered, and her jaws began moving, as she bit up and down uncontrollably, with the same unworldly quickness.

"Jesus!" I exclaimed. "How long can this go on?"

"Who knows?" Rind said. "It can take the body a while to adjust."

"How long is that?" I asked. "Hours?"

"Sometimes, it takes days," he said.

"Days?!" I responded. "Can the body take it?"

"It knows to stop and rest when the person gets tired," he said.

Her jaws began biting in all directions.

"She's going to crack her teeth!" I exclaimed.

"No," Rind responded. "The body knows to adjust for things like that. It isn't going to do things to injure itself."

We helped Liz onto the exam table. The 'reacquainting process' continued, progressing from the muscles of the head downward. The pattern was always the same: It began a shock wave ripped through her body, and heralded the movement of the reacquainting process in a new muscle group. Then, the movements began.

The process followed a seemingly orderly progression, sequentially moving from the muscles of her neck, to her shoulders, back, arms and legs. The movements were too fast to be voluntary, and seemingly too precise to be involuntary.

It was apparently as Dr. Rind had described – The brain was reacquainting itself with each individual muscle fiber; familiarizing itself with the muscle's every action and movement for the first time; learning the correct circuits to voluntarily operate the muscles all over again.

At times, the movements seemed violent, as the muscles stretched the limbs to the extent of their capability. It also seemed like certain muscle groups were receiving more attention than others, particularly those involved in movement of the eyes, jaws, neck and thumbs. At other times, Liz's body seemed to twist and assume odd positions, as it readied itself for another reacquainting session.

"Here we go again," she said.

Her left shoulder began contorting – The rapidity and containment of the gyrations suggested something beyond voluntary control. Then, her left foot – First, at the ankle, then at the great toe. Ultimately, it moved to the hip. It had the effect of looking like Liz were a marionette, being pulled back and forth by strings.

I turned to Dr. Rind.

"Were you focusing on certain muscles when you worked on her?" I asked.

"No," he said. "I just found the restriction in her temporal bone and relieved it. After that, her body's been in control."

"And correcting that one little bone is responsible for all this?"

"To my mind it's not a minor maneuver," he responded. "If my car doesn't start, it's because there's a bad connection between the ignition and the battery. Someone who knows what to do can just come in and knock on the turbo, and the next thing you know, the car can start. But if you don't understand what's going on, then it's a miraculous event. In other words, this whole system just got going because this man made a little tap. It's the same thing in Medicine. Her whole brain, her whole body, her whole nervous system – Everything just got kicked into place because that 'one little bone' was impeding the good function of the brain. Now, suddenly, it's no longer an issue and the brain can function. So it looks like miraculous things are happening, but it's really nothing more than basic physiology, if you apply these principles. You see what I'm saying?..." •

Between contortions, her body stayed still for a long time. I didn't know whether it was because the subconscious was integrating what it had just experienced, or if it was scanning the body for the next distinct set of muscles it wanted to initiate into the reacquainting process? Her body moved her like an automaton. It was like her subconscious was connecting to a new set of circuits and looking for the best way to master the gears...

Assisting Liz off the exam table, she described feeling changed.

"It's like getting use to a complete re-wiring job," she said. "With each step, though, I'm more familiar with how the limb works."

Dr. Rind checked her reflexes again.

"All her reflexes are bilaterally symmetrical and normal," he said.

"No?" I thought. "It can't be."

Taking the reflex hammer, I repeated the examination – Her reflexes were indeed equal!

"I feel like I'm being held up by puffs of air," Liz declared. "At my back, my front, by my sides. I feel like my mind hasn't connected with my muscles yet..."

CHAPTER THIRTY

Elizabeth called from her apartment.

"Mike, something's happening," she said.

Her mother had since returned to Rhode Island, so I hurried over to check on her.

Arriving at the apartment, Liz was on the couch, undergoing movements similar to those at Dr. Rind's clinic – except (this time) her arm was contracting back-and-forth, so to propel her hand against her upper chest.

"What is it, Mike?" she asked.

"You're beating on your thymus," I said. "According to Chinese Medicine, it's the organ that's supposed to represent the center of the life force."

She looked into the distance.

"For the past days I've been on the verge of tears," she confided. "Like life was too much for me, and I wanted to just 'check out.' I wonder if this is my body's reaction?... To say, 'No, I'm going to force the life into you...'"

As the unwinding process continued, Liz displayed a flexibility that I wouldn't have thought possible.

"When I was young, I danced ballet," she explained. "I stopped to go into academics. Now, it's like my body is retaliating for not having danced in all those years..."

CHAPTER THIRTY-ONE

Dr. Rind asked me to assist with a Bioenergy class he was teaching for patients and medical providers. Included in those present was Dr. Eskinazi from the Office of Alternative Medicine.

"I want to start by reading a passage from a book by Brian Brooks," Rind began. "He writes, 'What I've learned from my experience is that the most important part of healing is the giving of unconditional love.' If I impart anything to you today, I hope that will be part of it..."

Dr. Rind demonstrated Bioenergy: Selecting a woman in the front row, he scanned her and determined an energy imbalance in her hip.

"Mike, come up here and release the strain at the joint," he said.

Energy radiated from her hip. It was slow to release, though, and thinking that those in attendance might get bored, and not wanting to delay the class, I hurried through it, without applying the exacting pursuit of the energy's path that I usually performed.

"Let's see," Dr. Rind said.

He tested her range of motion. It was better, but still restricted.

"Wait a minute," he declared.

He followed the strain in three dimensions, then tested it again. A hush ran through the crowd as he demonstrated significantly improved range of motion.

"The demonstration was very important to me," the woman said. "It showed how different styles and levels of experience contribute to healing."

Dr. Rind chose another participant, then turned to me.

"Mike, Melissa has a number of energy vectors all over her," he said. "Let's work on neutralizing them together."

Dr. Rind stood still and followed the energy in three dimensions; I, meanwhile, followed the path of energy arising from her in wide panoramic movements, as I traced the elliptical orbit of the energy.

"It was very different," Melissa said. "I see auras, and what I saw was very different when the two of you worked on me separately, and then combined."

Dr. Eskinazi raised his hand.

"How far away can you be from the person you're healing and still achieve an effect?" he asked. "Could you heal someone from the other side of a telephone line?"

"I don't know," Dr. Rind responded. "Let's see."

Dr. Rind invited Dr. Eskinazi to sit in the front, determined a focus of strain Dr. Eskinazi's hip, and demonstrated the resultant limitation in motion. Then, Dr. Rind turned to me.

"Mike, go to the other side of the hall," he instructed, "get in one of the examining rooms and when I call to you, focus your thought on the lesion."

In the other room I waited for Dr. Rind's signal. In the meantime, he demonstrated Eskinazi's limitation of motion for a second time.

"Okay, Mike," he called to me. "You can think now."

Through the laughter that momentarily filled the room, I focused my thoughts on Dr. Eskinazi's hip, visualizing in my mind the normal anatomy. Just then, around the corner, gasps erupted from the larger room; and making my way to the doorway, I looked in and watched Dr. Rind demonstrate full range of motion in Eskinazi's leg…

CHAPTER THIRTY-TWO

"I had an interesting experience with one of the people in Dr. Rind's class," I told Liz. "I'd been feeling for energy over her head when I developed a sensation of tightness over my eyes. When I asked her, she said that she was having problems with sinus headaches. It was as though I was interlinking with her without touching her."

"Why don't you try it on me?" Liz said.

She put out her hand. As I scanned over it, I experienced a feeling of tightness in my lower abdomen.

"I know," she said. "I'm having my period."

Opening myself to the feeling, I experienced wave after wave of energy.

"It was the same for me," Liz said. "First, down to my feet. Then, a dramatic shift, up to my head."

"All the time that you were working on me," she continued, "I had no pain. Not until the moment you took your hands away. Then, the pain returned."

She smiled.

"I think that you should continue on the alternative medicine path," she said. "One day you might be very good and help many people. I think that it's important that you have this time. Right now, you carry too much arrogance. It's because of fear and low self-esteem. You're too hard on people."

I shook my head.

"I do it to protect myself," I confided.

"That's the point," she said. "One day you won't feel that way, and then you'll be able to help many more people..."

CHAPTER THIRTY-THREE

Shortly after accompanying Dr. Rind into the exam room of a woman with neck pain, he was called out to attend another patient.

"Mike, why don't you work with Evelyn doing Bioenergy till I get back?" he suggested.

As he left the room, I smiled.

"Has Dr. Rind ever done Bioenergy with you before?" I asked.

"No," she responded, nervously. "I don't think so. What is that?"

"It's an energy medicine technique," I responded. "It involves scanning the body for energy disturbances and then neutralizing them to help the body recover function. Would you like to try?"

"I guess so," she replied, doubtfully.

I positioned myself to her side and scanned her energetically.

"I don't feel anything," she commented, anxiously.

But I did. I was a strange, uncomfortable buzz inside my system, like having a paralyzing headache.

"Okay," I responded, endeavoring to maintain my composure. "Why don't we wait for Dr. Rind?"

I went to the door and slowly left the room.

Then – unable to shake the feeling – I left the clinic.

Later that day I visited Liz.

"Mike, would you do some Bioenergy on my back?" she asked, rubbing her sides. "It's been bothering me all day."

Scanning her from behind, she smiled.

"I think that I can feel where your hand is," she said.

I depressed the corners of my lips.

"Where is it?" I asked.

"It's at my shoulder," she said.

"Which shoulder?" I asked.

"The right one," she responded, correctly.

I moved it somewhere else.

"Now it's at my sacrum," she asserted.

I moved it again.

"Where is it now?" I asked.

"At my head," she said. "I can feel the energy coming from it. That's amazing."

Amazed, I stepped back – Tears spontaneously welling in my eyes.

She turned.

"Why are you crying?" she asked.

"Because I cherish you so much," I said.

I let out a deep breath.

"For the past weeks I haven't known exactly what to do," I continued. "It doesn't seem like you're getting better. You're losing weight again. I don't know what to do."

"Mike, this is the happiest that I've been in years."

But as I scanned her again, a spreading feeling of tightness expanded across my chest.

"Liz, I'm having a problem," I confided. "I'm experiencing chest pain."

I sat.

"This isn't the first time this has happened," I continued. "There have been other times, as well – Where I'm working on a patient, and I get this funny buzz... It's like an uncomfortable feeling. And usually, when it happens, I'm not able to help the person... The Bioenergy isn't doing anything for them, and I'm left standing there, embarrassed."

I shook my head, slouched in the chair, then crossed my arms and looked away.

"I don't think I can do this anymore, Liz," I lamented. "I don't think I can do Bioenergy... I don't like this feeling. Sometimes it stays with me all day."

"I don't think what's happening is anything that your patients are 'doing' to you," Liz commented. "They're not hurting you in any way. I think that when you treat them, it's bringing out wounds buried deep within you. I imagine for the most part they're lying under the surface where you usually can't see or feel them, because you've suppressed them a long time ago. But they're still there, unresolved and waiting for you to come to terms with them."

"I think that these patients who are making you 'feel bad' are just somehow bringing these unresolved wounds to the surface," she continued. "You can't help these patients until you resolve these injuries in you. The 'buzz' that you're feeling is probably your body making you aware of them and giving you a chance to heal them."

"But how?" I asked, doubtfully.

"I think a form of self-healing might help you," she answered, matter-of-factly. "Maybe you should try Chi Gong?"

"What's that?"

"It's a form of Chinese healing," she responded. "It's a lot like Bioenergy, but it's *self-healing* – like meditation."

"A local Chi Gong group is sponsoring an outreach lecture this weekend," she added. "The Master is flying in from Taiwan. We should go..."

CHAPTER THIRTY-FOUR

At the Newton High School Liz and I sat waiting for the lecture to begin. Looking around the auditorium, it appeared we were the only Caucasians in attendance and everyone else was Asian. Then, a tall Asian man tood the stage with a shorter man beside him.

"I'm Paul Mok, senior assistant for our True Nature Chi Gong group," said the shorter man. "I will translate for Master Chou for the English speakers in the audience."

Master Chou spoke in Chinese.

"First, the Master welcomes all the newcomers," Paul translated.

Master Chou spoke again.

"The Master would like to know if any of the newcomers has ever practiced Chi Gong or something similar?"

Recalling that Liz suggested that Chi Gong was similar to Bioenergy, I raised my hand.

The Master looked in my direction, then spoke to the interpreter.

"The Master would like to know your definition of Chi Gong?" Paul directed to me.

I stood.

"It's a matter of tapping into a certain universal energetic blueprint from which all things are derived," I said, "and channeling that information to help heal unreconciled wounds."

The Master nodded, as though genuinely impressed, and spoke to the interpreter.

"That is a good definition," Paul declared.

The Master spoke again.

"Chi is the life force," Paul translated. "The Universal Chi runs through all things. Trauma severs our connection with the life force. To restore the Gong, which can be translated as 'function', we have to remedy the source of trauma. This we do through the practice of Chi Gong."

"He's talking about healing at the level of the primary lesion," I thought.

"By ridding the body of trauma," Paul continued, translating, "we eliminate those things that stood in the way of our being fully natural. In this way, Chi Gong restores us to our true selves."

"'Fully natural'?" I thought. "Is he talking about remedying the psyche?"

I raised my hand again. The Master nodded in acknowledgement.

"Does Chi Gong work for emotional as well as physical trauma?" I asked.

This time the Master answered himself.

"It works for all trauma," he asserted...

CHAPTER THIRTY-FIVE

After the lecture, a friendly-looking but professional-sounding Asian American man approached me, saying he was a representative of the Chi Gong group.

"Hi, I'm Albert," he said. "I'm the Secretary for the group. I've been doing Chi Gong for about five years. Master Chou was very impressed with your answers to his question. He'd like you to know if you'd be interested in joining the group."

"Yes, I would be interested," I said. "Does it involve much?"

"Master Chou asks that members follow a dress code," he said. "He says it's like you're attending a formal ceremony, and wearing a white top and black bottoms is a sign of respect, as if you're stepping into an ancient classroom to receive the dharma."

"What is 'dharma'?" I asked.

"Dharmas are 'teachings'," he answered. "They're the energetic encapsulation of Master Chou's cultivation and practice. Listening to his teachings transmits the dharmas to you, so that you can benefit from the Master's experience."

"Anyway, I'll talk with some of the other members," he concluded, "and we'll plan to get back to you..."

CHAPTER THIRTY-SIX

The following day, Albert reached out to me again.

"The Master would like you to join our group," he said. "He told us that he thought you learned Chi Gong from this doctor who you studied with, but your platform is just on the physical being of a person, and not addressing the spiritual body, and without that, you're not realizing your life's mission – What you can bring to people around you – and reach the full capacity of what your life's mission is. And you can't reach that capacity if you're just using chi to make better health for people; it will only happen if you progress spiritually."

"It's not a criticism," he added. "And your life mission can be simple. It could be to make your home a safe harbor for everybody you meet - Your friends, strangers - But you can't do it alone. You have to achieve that with the group. You have to come to the group to receive the benefit."

"And you will feel the difference," he concluded. "Because you're very sensitive. We can all see that..."

I met Albert back at the high school. There, he handed me a paper with some typed instructions.

"This is a list of Chi Gong requirements," he said.

Chi Gong Prerequisites.
1. Complete vegetarian diet without garlic or onions or leeks.
2. No addictions including cigarette smoking, alcohol consumption or gambling.
3. No restriction on milk or eggs, although limiting consumption of these is recommended because, at least eggs, clog the thoughts

and produces impurities in the spirit.

4. Cleansing of the mouth (no insults or foul language), and no negative intentions ("internal thunder").

5. Keep a Chi Gong diary of negative thoughts.

6. Vow to help others in the world.

7. Vow to be united as one in future cultivation.

Reading through the list, I nodded.

"I can abide by these," I said.

Albert led me to the gymnasium, where the lights were low and the group had gathered. All of them appeared Asian.

"Master Chou will initiate you into the chi field," he said. "First, though, he wanted us to prepare you. We're going to line up, and when we say, 'Ey', stand up straight and fill your body with energy. When we say 'Chi', that's the signal to bow."

"I'm prohibited from bowing," I said, "as a matter of my religion."

"Only do what you feel comfortable with," he responded. "We understand that people from some faiths don't want to do that. For us, it's just a sign of respect. Keep in mind, though, we don't bow all the way to the ground – We bow only to the level of the spirit heart, so, really, you're bowing to yourself. You can hold your hands outwards palms up at about the level of your hips, or you can overlap your hands over your spirit heart. Standing that way will help you reach a state of stability. I'm sure you felt that before in the work you do with the doctor you spoke of.

"At some point you'll feel like your energy connects with the energy of the universe, and you'll start moving. Let the chi enter your body and move you wherever it wants to go."

I looked at him, confused.

"How will I know that the chi has entered my body?" I asked. "What will I feel?"

"For me, most of the time, the energy comes from the bottom of my feet, like it's bubbling up. It's like electricity, but also like warm spring water that rises. And the bubbles are like a very fine champagne – Real small, but a lot of them. Then, I start moving. Sometimes, Master Chou teaches to start by stamping your feet, and that way the energy comes from your axis – from the inside of you – to initiate the movement. That's why we call it 'True nature' Chi Gong."

"How does energy initiate movement?" I asked. "Does it act at the muscles?"

"Even before I was initiated, when I met Master Chou and saw the others practicing, I felt this energy pull my ankle and make me turn around in a circle," he said. "I spun in a circle. And I knew that the energy for that was coming from the group."

"And it takes control of your body?" I asked.

"Uh-huh, yes," he responded. "I let it go."

"I've only felt energy at my hands," I said. "Do you ever feel it there?"

"Yeah, sometimes my hands will feel real warm, like they're tingling," he responded.

Just then, Master Chou appeared and took his place in the front of the group, standing alongside Paul. The other members assembled, standing in well-formed rows and columns, and an older, balding man stepped forward to the front row.

"Ey," the older man called out, and even I experienced it like a summons to attention. "First bow – Be grateful for the energy of the universe. Chi... Second bow – Be grateful for the instruction from our teacher. Chi... Third bow, be grateful for the support from our Chi-mates. Chi... Fourth bow, be grateful and return the fruits of our laborers to the universe..."

I stood attempting to open myself to connecting energetically with the Universal Chi. My eyes closed, I could feel movement around me, as members of the group seemed to peeled off, with trotting feet that seemed to run all around the gymnasium.

Closing my eyes, I experienced energy radiating from my palms. The energy directed my hands upwards, and I followed the energy until it led me into a spin like a windmill in the wind.

My acceleration increased till I thought at any moment I would lose control and tumble and fall to the ground; instead, though, I experienced some internal release at the level of my chest, and an inner feeling of elation, like some joy bursting forth from me.

Opening my eyes, I found that Master Chou was "dancing" around me. Viewing him this way, in the sparsely lit room and myself still spinning, it was like watching someone being illuminated by a strobe light, so that as I spun and he continued to circle me, I saw what looked akin to still-shots of his movements, which resembled poses of something like a powerful Native American warrior dancing about a fire...

CHAPTER THIRTY-SEVEN

April and I attended a Peace Benefit featuring a prominent Israeli singer and well-known Palestinian activist named David Broza.

"I met David before," April said. "He told me that Israel is a hard place to leave. He said, 'You can go out of Israel, but Israel doesn't go out of you.'"

"It was very difficult when he left Israel," she continued. "My family was still living in Israel then, and David had been the country's favorite singer. On the kibbutz we sang all of his songs. They were beautiful.

"When David left the country, the press published pictures of him drunk in America. We were ashamed. When I asked him, he said that he couldn't stay in Israel because of the policies against the Palestinians - it was too much for him..."

We sat in the front row and enjoyed the music. After Broza played, a number of speakers assembled and debated the question of the occupied territories. The Palestinian representative painted a bleak picture, saying "the settlers and the Israeli government have created a nightmare for millions of Palestinians."

"Occupation is a de-humanizing experience for all involved," he continued. "It is demeaning for the occupied as well as the occupier - the victor and the vanquished.

"Learning cruelty is intrinsic to the trade of occupation. The occupiers emerge as not just tormentors, but, also, victims, who take out their frustrations on the even more abject and powerless captives under their supervision and control."

Then, he looked out at us, unblinking, and spoke with a force that only moral authority could supply.

"Shut away in the occupation is the ominous secret between us," he concluded. "That we are not enemies, but brothers…"

CHAPTER THIRTY-EIGHT

Leaving the Benefit, April and I walked to the car. Another couple (with an infant and two daughters) were parked nearby. Their infant was crying, and as the woman struggled to console the child, the man threw up his arms and slammed them against the car, while his two daughters stood cowering and looking about, uncertain.

"That's how my father was with us," I confided. "He was always upset."

We drove to a night club.

"How did you get interested in archeology, April?" I asked.

"The kibbutz where I grew up was built on top of an old Phoenician burial ground," she said. "All the tombs had been dug up earlier by the British, and only the empty hollows remained. I would go into the hollows and hide when I was a little girl. It was one of my many escapes from the other kibbutzniks that didn't like me."

"I was one of the un-liked kids who was looked down on by everyone," she continued. "In the kibbutz it's like that. You have the children that are adored by everyone, and others who are scorn.

"My sister was liked by everyone - she could do no wrong. It seemed like I couldn't do anything right, no matter what I did."

"My favorite uncle died there last year," she confided. "The family kept it hush-hush - I think because he had AIDS. I never had the chance to tell him how much I loved him because, when I finally did find out, he was too far gone, and died alone without me ever able to tell him my feelings for him."

I nodded.

"My grandmother died alone," I said. "When I told my father that I wanted to visit her, he said, 'What would visiting her do?... You're not gonna cure her.' He said that when he finally went to see her in the hospital, he didn't recognize her. 'I could not believe that the woman in that room was my mother,' he said. 'If I hadn't seen the number on the door - if I hadn't seen the name on the chart - I wouldn't have known that that was my mother."

"My mother suffers from depression," I continued. "A month ago my father called and told me that I had to commit myself to taking care of her. 'You only have one mother,' he said. 'You have to make a commitment. You can say anything that you like, but she's the only mother that you've got. You've got to make a commitment. Sure, I wasn't always there for my mother. I had lots of excuses. There was work and making money? Would I do things differently if I had it to do all over again? Yes. If I had it all to do over again, I would have taken better care of my mother. Because you only have one. That's why you have to make a commitment. If your mother's important to you, then you'll get down here and take care of her. You'll make a commitment...'"

"Oh, sure," April interrupted. "So, you're supposed to quit school, quit work and go back home."

I looked into the distance.

"When I was in Israel," I said, "my father made a stop-over and stayed with me for a few days. At the time I was heartbroken. I wanted to talk to him because I'd put my faith in things that he had told me. He'd said that I'd be happier when I got into medical school and would find somebody else. When I told him how much I missed her, he said, 'Look, when it comes to relationships, you go out with a few girls, here and there, and when you get tired of all that, you marry someone. You just get tired of that kind of thing after a while. You get lonely, so you settle down, and that's what happens.'

"I remember listening and experiencing this feeling of utter disbelief. 'You get lonely?' I thought. 'Are you kidding?' I felt like someone had just pulled the biggest practical joke on me in the world."

April sank into the car seat and looked away.

"Sometimes that's the hand you're dealt," she uttered.

An awkward silence followed.

I've ruined the evening, I thought. I wonder if I shouldn't ask if she'd just like to go home?

But arriving at the club, rather than dispirited, April appeared anxious to go inside. Following her to the dancefloor, she lost herself in the music, looking in harmony with everything around her as she danced. It was as though she'd cast away some shroud that had been covering her; letting go of past sadness; and choosing, instead, to engage and embrace life.

As a round of slow songs started, she took my hand and pulled me to the bar.

"Have you ever had Arak?" she asked. "It's a licorice liqueur made from the Chimiele plant. We used to grow it on the kibbutz. I remember sucking on it when I was little."

She gazed out.

"I like this place," she said.

Not long after returning to the dancefloor, a second round of slow songs began. She looked at me.

"Well?" she asked.

Pulling her close, I perceived contractions darting from her solar plexus, and holding her, it felt as though her ribs were tightly packed.

"She carries a lot of sadness," I thought. "Like me."

Then, she laid her head on my shoulder and draped herself around me...

CHAPTER THIRTY-NINE

At the next meeting of the Chi Gong group I was greeted by Master Chou's main assistant and interpreter, Paul.

"The Master is leaving," he said. "He is flying to Philadelphia tonight to be with the group up there. So, he told us to guide you during your chi cultivation period."

"What is the cultivation period?" I asked.

"It is a time when you will awaken your chi," he responded. "The Master said your original energy is very pure. Now, your chi is weak and unbalanced. The reason it's not as strong now is because of all the things that you have experienced in life. So, now, we want to help you go back to your pure state - Your primary spirit - Your true nature.

"All of us are connected to the Universal Chi. In the next weeks you will participate in practices with the group that are meant to bring chi into your body and store it. It will bring you back into harmony with the chi and supply you with the healing energy that you can call on in times of illness."

He guided me to the older man, who was the one who called out the commands for the preparatory bows.

"Now, I want to introduce you to one of our senior members," Paul said. "This is Wah Lee. Wah is a physicist. He works at the Food and Drug Administration. We thought that because you are both scientists, Wah would be a good choice for the person to supervise you during your chi cultivation period."

Wah shook my hand and seemed to study me, smiling amused.

"Your body thinks that the norm is a state of total stress," he said with a stutter. "I can see it in the way that you hold your shoulders. Your back is all twisted, too. We have to reset your thermostat back to its original true nature. I can do some 'Healing Hands' on you and try to open up your blockages. Most blockages are because of a lack of circulation of energy. Others think it's nerves or a circulation problem, but when someone does Healing Hands on you, sometimes that can unblock it. If you like, I can do that for you."

I shrugged.

"I'd be interested," I said.

Positioning himself behind me, Wah closed his eyes. Then, his face lost all expression, and, suddenly, his arms contracted back and forth, till his hands met at my back. At first the pressure of the blows was gentle, performed with an open hand. Then, as he honed in on certain areas, he closed his fists and pounded till the breath was forced out of me. Throughout this process, he moved mechanically in utter silence, as though he'd been transformed into some automaton – detached and completely focused on the task of healing. It struck me that Wah's movements were not unlike those displayed by Elizabeth when she underwent that neuromuscular re-education at Dr. Rind's clinic; and the effect of his movements was not unlike the percussion hammer that Dr. Rind used to treat his patients.

Could they be related? I thought. Was he connecting via some internal neural network with my energetic circulation, so to know how to *physically* help me, like a human medical instrument?

As my muscles relaxed, the rapidity of Wah's movements slowed; then, he held me till my heart rate quieted, and I experienced a sense of being entirely clear thinking.

"How do you feel?" Wah asked, standing in front of me again and resuming his former smiling, jocular manner.

Turning from side to side, I encountered none of the usual resistance in my back muscles.

"Better," I responded. "I can move easier, like you ironed out the kinks in my system. How did you do that?"

"I put myself in a Chi Gong state and asked the universal chi to let me work on you," he responded.

"So, you weren't consciously aware of what you were doing?" I asked.

"No," he replied, assertively. "I let the chi guide me."

"Will I be able to do that?" I asked.

"You have to complete your cultivation period first," he declared. "After that, we'll see if you train as an assistant…"

CHAPTER FORTY

On Friday evening I met April at the Smithsonian Building. Climbing to the rooftop, we looked out at the DC skyline.

"I'm transferring to New York," she confided. "I was accepted for an internship there. I'll be working on a restoration project at the Metropolitan Museum."

I nodded.

"I'll miss you," I responded, blankly.

"Will I see you?" she asked.

I shrugged.

"I always want to see you," I replied.

Turning so she couldn't see me, I grimaced.

What is wrong with me? I thought. Why am I only able to offer these vague remarks?

She looked at me.

"Do you have a girlfriend, Michael?"

"Yeah," I admitted, doubtful. "She's more like something of a guide in my spiritual journey. And I think she needs me now..."

CHAPTER FORTY-ONE

"We can only be friends," I told April.

Standing naked under a shower of running water, I kissed her.

Then, suddenly, I found myself alone, wondering if Liz would discover us? And how stupid I'd been!...

"That's why she left!" Liz responded, laughing, despite my hardly having told her the contents of the dream. "She left because you didn't want to get into any more trouble. We like to think that our dreams represent all of our suppressed wishes and that we get them all out in our dreams, but it turns out that even in our dreams our desires are complicated by our conscience, and even there we can't do exactly what we'd wish."

"I don't deliberately want to let you go," she added. "When you become mature, you'll leave on your own. So why force the issue?..."

CHAPTER FORTY-TWO

At a Thanksgiving banquet I overheard a guest comment about me in passing.

"He mimics what he wants to do," she remarked, "and what his parents want him to do, and doesn't live at all..."

Awakening from the dream, I gazed at Liz. Her figure was fuller now, and I had difficulty reconciling the voluptuous woman who I was holding with the memory in my head.

She told me that she'd been this way before her illness, but I hadn't believed her or imagined it could be true...

"When I hold you," she said, "I experience a feeling of joy and friendship - like we were children, playing on a sunny day in an open field. It's an almost mystical feeling. When I meditate, I see an image of you - you're always naked, sitting in a lotus position; there are swirls of energy about you, and you either have your eyes closed, or you're smiling at me with your brightest smile. It's this image that my eyes call to mind before I can smile into the rest of my body. And, in the times that I'll be upset and won't be able to find my way and feel like there's something that I've forgotten, I'll call up your image and be able to move forward again."

She turned.

"Michael, do you still think I have a funny smile?"

"Why do you say that?" I replied, taken aback and confused and not understanding at all the basis for her asking.

"Because, that first time I met you in the clinic, you said that my upper lip appeared different somehow. Later, you asked Dr. Weber about it, and he said it was because of the faulty way that I used my jaw in order to accommodate a misalignment in my bite."

Tears formed in my eyes.

"No," I said. "I don't think you smile funny anymore."

"Why are you crying?" she asked.

"Because when we first met," I said, "it seemed like nothing came natural for you, and everything was forced - even your smile. And, now, it isn't that way anymore."

I find you truly beautiful, I thought.

"Everything had been an effort before," she said. "When you're sick, everything is."

She hesitated.

"I remember the first time you came to my apartment," she said. "I was sitting all bunched up, with my knees to my chest on one end of the couch. I hoped you would sit at the other end and, naturally, you sat in the middle, which made me bunch up even more. And how surprised I felt when you kissed me, because I thought that I was old and unattractive and sick."

She looked at me.

"Michael, do you believe I love you?"

I shrugged.

"I know you love me," I responded, matter-of-factly.

"I remember the day I went to your place," she began. "You pulled me close and held me. There had always been a pain in my chest. I'd always had it. It's just a little pain, but it's always there, even to this day. It goes away the instant that my chest makes contact with yours, just as it did that first day..."

CHAPTER FORTY-THREE

At the Glen Echo Park, Liz and I signed up for lessons in ballroom dancing.

Liz was happy and excited.

"Like this, Miker," she instructed, smiling.

I shook my head.

"It's difficult - this swing and waltzing," I confided. "I get frustrated."

"You should think about it like making love," Liz said. "Like you're tossing and turning with me the same as we do in bed, only standing."

"Liz, you're making me laugh," I said.

"Why am I making you laugh, Miker?"

"Because you're leading again," I responded.

"I remember when you used to come over to my apartment," she said. "You'd laugh so hard at the things I'd say that you'd have to excuse yourself. 'Excuse me,' you'd say. You always said it so softly."

She laughed.

"You could have just asked me to stop," she said. "I would have, you know."

I looked at her.

"I don't think that I really wanted you to," I said...

After the dance lesson Liz and I strolled outside about the garden.

"Do you think you've changed?" she asked.

I shook my head.

"You have," she asserted. "You've become calmer - more tranquil, less intense."

"That isn't because of any change in me," I said. "It's because of the friends who surround me now."

"Friends make all the difference," she affirmed, "because they help you and give you a chance to practice and cultivate the elements inside of you."

We sat on a bench.

"Mike, what did you feel the first time that you held me?"

"I don't remember," I said.

She looked away.

"I thought that I was a bag of bones," she said. "It was the skinniest I'd ever been."

I nodded.

"I was just afraid for your health," I said.

"The first time that we made love," she continued, "I had the sensation of being surrounded by flowers - and that sensation was very funny, because whenever I opened my eyes, I'd find myself in your decrepit little room in the Cloister. But, still, I couldn't get the sensation of being surrounded by flowers out of my mind."

She looked out at the garden. It was the beginning of spring, and the plants and flowers were in different stages of bloom.

"Mike, do you think that you can feel the energy coming off of plants?" she asked.

"I don't think so, Liz?"

"Have you ever tried?"

"No, I never thought of it?"

"Why don't you, then?"

I scanned the flowers.

"That's interesting," I said. "I do feel something."

Flowers with larger trumpets gave off more energy than smaller more delicate flowers; trees with more grooves and bark had more energy than those with smooth outsides; leaves with smooth edges radiated less energy than ruffled ones; plants with spines emitted an feeling of pins and needles, whereas ferns produced a tickling sensation.

"It's as though the shape of the plant follows the energy somehow," I said. "Energy defines morphology - It serves as a blueprint that directs the plants growth."

"Feel this, Miker," she said.

She had her hand over a bud about to flower. Guiding my hand over it, the energy speared my palm, like an arrow through it.

"None of the others felt like this," she said.

"Probably because they've already flowered," I said. "Their potential has been reached. This one's still working on what it's about to become."

Coming upon a tree with a large tumorous growth on its trunk, Liz scanned it, then looked at me, surprised.

"The growth has no energy," she said.

"Probably because a tumor has no blueprint for morphology," I said. "It's just a randomly growing mass. It has no direction, so no energy."

Liz turned to me and hugged me and told me that she loved me.

"I like to play with you wherever we go," she said. "I always want to be your playmate..."

CHAPTER FORTY-FOUR

Arriving back at the apartment, Liz's friend, Marie, was holding her infant son, Roland.

"Roland has another ear infection," Marie said. "We just came back from the doctors. He wants to insert tubes."

Elizabeth turned to me.

"Mike," she said, "is there something that you could do."

I shrugged.

"I could try," I said.

I scanned the infant.

"There are these huge surges of energy coming from behind the ears," I said. "It's really intense. When he turns his head, it's like being hit by a spray of electric particles…"

Later that evening, Liz looked in on Marie and Roland.

"Marie said Roland stopped crying shortly after you worked on him," Liz related, "so she was able to put him to bed…"

CHAPTER FORTY-FIVE

Liz found a new acupuncturist and wanted to introduce me.

"Dr. Shou is also a renown Chi Gong Master," she said. "He's been serving as a Traditional Chinese Medicine expert on President Clinton's Executive Committee on Alternative Medicine. I thought it would be good for you to meet him…"

Dr. Shou's Office wasn't far from the Georgetown Medical School, where I was performing my graduate studies. The inside was small and pleasantly lit, with a couple exam rooms, in which he cared for patients.

"How you get interested in Chi Gong?" Dr. Shou asked in broken English.

"I hurt my leg about a year ago," I said. "Conventional treatments didn't help, so I sought other forms of healing."

Dr. Shou indicated that he wanted to examine my leg and passed his hand over me.

"Feel very warm," he said. "Means lots of chi."

Then, he excused himself.

"Treated patient with bad kidney," he said. "Now, feel bad at kidney."

He turned, but I called to him.

"Dr. Shou, I've trained in a technique called Bioenergy," I said. "It's a way of removing energy strains. May I try it on you?"

He accepted. Scanning him, I perceived an energy disturbance in his mid-back. Following it, the energy strain released within seconds.

"Your technique very good," he said. "Move energy well. Have to take care, though. Bad energy from others get into your body. Make you sick like them."

Then, he turned from side to side, nodding his head.

"Your chi very good," he said. "All discomfort gone."

"Still, have to take care," he continued. "Do not want you practice chi. Too much risk for you. Your muscles still too weak. Cannot take strain of giving your chi to others."

"I don't give my chi to others," I said. "I merely act as a conduit for the universal life force to move through me."

"Maybe true," he responded, "but always risk that your energy come out with it. Current flow down river with least resistance. First need to cultivate chi..."

CHAPTER FORTY-SIX

Paul led the Chi Gong group in its preparatory bows before initiating the practice.

"Begin," he said.

As the practice commenced, energy flowed into my hands. Then, something odd happened: My body was physically moved, so that it felt like some force had taken hold of me, and my movement was outside of my conscious control.

The movement was light and completely unlabored, as though walking on air. It was like nothing that I'd ever experienced, because, this time, I wasn't following the energy, but, rather, the energy was directing me.

"It was just a few short steps," I told Wah at the conclusion of practice, "but it felt like the most extraordinary journey of my life."

"I'm happy for you, Mike," he said. "That's what Chi Gong is supposed to feel like. Some practice for a life time and never experience that…"

CHAPTER FORTY-SEVEN

Paul pulled me aside.

"Master Chou has chosen you to become an assistant," he said. "Though you haven't been practicing Chi Gong for very long, he thinks, in your heart, there are all the qualifications to be an assistant."

He smiled, broadly.

"Congratulations," he continued. "This is a big honor."

I was taken aback and didn't know how to respond.

"What do you see as your mission in life?" he asked.

"I want to continue my Bioenergy training with Dr. Rind," I said, "and cultivate my ability to serve as a channel for healing - a conduit for correcting energy imbalances."

"Through Chi Gong," he responded, "you will become an energy conductor... A deliverer of that energy."

"I don't know that I want that," I replied. "It sounds forceful. I just want to help others reconcile their energy blockages. That's why I entered Chi Gong - so that I could rid myself of the blockages that were getting in the way of being a better healer."

"How successful have you been with curing patients using Bioenergy?" he queried.

"I've had many successes," I said, "but, also, failures."

"What failures?" Paul asked.

I lifted my brow.

"Elizabeth, for example," I said.

"Why do you think that you haven't been able to help her?" he asked.

"Two reasons," I replied. "Me and Liz."

"It's because of emotion," he said. "Emotions get in the way."

I nodded.

"It makes me wonder if I should do as Master Chou once told me?" I commented.

"What was that?" he asked.

"Limit my practice of Bioenergy till I rid myself of my imbalances," I said.

"I am pleased that you have come to that realization by yourself," he responded...

"I don't agree with that," Liz retorted when I shared the contents of my conversation with Paul. "I think your Bioenergy work with people has been very helpful. Look at what you were able to do for Marie's baby, Roland – He was having ear infections all the time. Since you worked on him that day, he hasn't had one."

"I want you to be able to go on helping others," she continued. "I understand how important it is to you to rid yourself of your imbalances. I mean, my last visit to Dr. Rind I wasn't satisfied because of his moodiness. He needs to work on that – But that doesn't mean that he should close his practice. You have to do the two things at the same time..."

CHAPTER FORTY-EIGHT

At the National Institutes of Health, the first patient in our cancer vaccine trial flew in from Texas.

"I'm John Swepstone," he said. "I play tennis with your collaborator, Tom Dinna. I guess he does the genetics for you before you came up with the vaccine. When he found out that I had pancreatic cancer, he invited me to take part in the study."

He shook my hand.

"I know how hard you've worked on this," he told me. "I can appreciate anyone who puts in eighty hours a week..."

"Talking to him the patient," I told Wah, "he said that he 'eats every bad thing he can get his hands on, drinks whiskey.' It left me feeling like, 'What's the point? Do you want to get better?'"

"People want a mechanic to fix them," Wah said. "They don't want to do the work."

I shook my head.

"Mike, what do you want to do now?" Wah said. "With your career, I mean."

"Perhaps, become a family practitioner," I said, "and use the skills that I've learned at Dr. Rind's clinic to help others."

"In that case, why do the PhD?"

"I want to see the project through," I said. "I can't help the feeling that I still have a reason for being here..."

A week later, a second patient was enrolled in the vaccine trial.

He was a dermatologist from Miami. Like our first patient, Dr. Hoffman also had pancreatic cancer.

"I read about your study in Newsweek," he said, "and decided to enroll."

He had a personable, business-like way about himself –
Pleasant, cordial, unassuming, not unlike my father.

But sitting in the wheelchair, his legs were swollen.

"His cancer must be very advanced," I thought.

His wife, Mrs. Hoffman, wore a worried expression.

"One day I can see your study doing much to help the indigent," she told me.

The couple's daughter was beautiful. She devotedly rubbed her mother's anxious shoulders.

I stood humbled in their presence...

CHAPTER FORTY-NINE

At the High School auditorium Paul delivered an outreach lecture about Chi Gong.

"I want to clarify some things about chi," he said. "When children are born, they possess 100% efficient and working chi. The chi is thought to have three components: the first is basic chi that sustains a baseline of normal function; the second is functional chi, which is there to permit better regulation should injury or trauma occur; the last is the undeveloped potential. This is the creative force that is unique for each person that can manifest in art, science, intuition or psychic sensitivity. Think about all of the amazing things that children do - they learn to walk, talk. Kids master these complex processes with no structured learning. It's purely a creative process. It's because they're making use of that 100% of chi. It's the creative component within the undeveloped potential that permits them to succeed in accomplish in the various stages of childhood on their own initiative for the most part..."

"A lot of conventional medicine is 'sweet poison,'" he said. "It makes you feel good, but it plays havoc on the body. It's like the old chi-chi joke. It goes like this. Three explorers get caught by tribe of aborigines. They're offered chi-chi or death. The first two pick chi-chi, and die terribly tortured deaths. The last says he's seen enough, and picks death. 'Death it is,' says the chieftain. 'But, first, a little chi-chi.'"

Those in attendance laughed, but Paul remained stoic.

"Sometimes, medicine is that way," Paul said. "The patient always dies, but the doctor gets to torture him a little first..."

CHAPTER FIFTY

Sitting in my mother's house, the phone rang. It was my brother.

"Just wanted to tell you that Liz was okay," he said. "Also, this just in: 'Researchers say Chi Gong unimaginable...'"

Awakening from the dream, I experienced a feeling of crushing pain in my chest.

Liz turned in bed.

"Miker, are you alright?" she asked.

"Yes, I'm okay," I responded, attempting to ignore it, as I changed my position.

She hesitated.

"Do an experiment for me," she said. "Move far away, then move closer."

She nodded.

"Yep, there's no doubt," she said. "I'm feeling a pain from you. The closer you get, the more I feel your vibrations and the worse the pain gets."

She held me, and I consider the source of the chest pain: Early in life, my uncle had struck me in the chest; it happened at the Metropolitan Museum; he'd coughed, and I patted his back to relieve him; then, something happened; it felt like the wind had been knocked out of me. I didn't feel any pain, but I had the feeling he might have 'thumped' me – hit me in the center of the chest with a closed fist.

"One day," Liz continued, "I want to make a fresco behind your bed of a blue night, with a moon and lots of stars for Miker to sleep with."

I laughed.

"I'm sorry, Liz," I said. "I had the image of counting sheep, with a cow leaping over the moon."

Liz lowered her head.

"When you laugh, it comes out like something hideous," she said. "Like you were deprived of that and don't know how to."

I stayed silent.

"You can't even imagine the thought of sleeping in a cute little, cuddly bed," she continued. "You never got to enjoy sweet cuddly things."

I smiled.

"Sorry, Liz, I was reminded of something," I explained. "When I was twelve, I received some money from my grandparents for my birthday. My mother took me to the toy store, and all I wanted was a mechanical toy dog."

I shook my head.

"Could you imagine?" I commented. "For a boy that age?"

"It's no crime to be sweet-natured the way you are," she responded. "You think so because that's what everyone told you... Maybe not directly, but that's the message they sent you."

"And what harm have you done to deserve such treatment?" she asked. "You're not looking to hurt anyone. You just want to be happy. It's who you are..."

CHAPTER FIFTY-ONE

My father called and described problems of ringing in his ears.

"The tinnitus is getting worse," he said. "I'm going to be in your area because a friend recommended that I see a specialist at Johns Hopkins."

"Why don't you come here, Dad?" I asked. "We could see what Dr. Rind thinks first, and then I'll take you to Johns Hopkins..."

My father and I met at a restaurant near the Metro Station. After the hostess seated us, he smiled broadly.

"So, how have you been doing, my son?" he said. "Have you learned anything new lately?"

"I've been studying a lot of alternative approaches to healing," I said. "I think that they're helping me - not just with the problem in the leg, but also my psyche."

"When it comes to that," he said, "the only important thing is that you recognize you have a problem and make efforts to do something about it."

"I think it requires more than that, Dad," I said. "You have to get to the root of it."

"I can appreciate that, Michael," he responded, "but really, I think you're wasting your time."

He shook his head.

"I mean, really, Michael, for the past year it's been really disappointing. Before it was like you always had a direction. Now I don't see that. I don't see any progress. You haven't written any papers, no big reports."

I lowered my gaze.

"How do you measure progress, Dad?" I asked.

"The yardstick I usually use is how much money you're making, or you're position in a job."

"Do you think you know what's best for me?"

"That doesn't matter," he said. "No matter what, I'm always going to push you to do more..."

After dinner we went to my apartment.

"So, Mike, what is that Dr. Rind going to do to me?" he asked, half-jokingly. "Is he going to do any of that 'Bioenergy' that you've been telling me about? What is that?"

"Bioenergy is the life force, Dad," I said. "What the Chinese call the chi. It emanates from everything."

He pointed to the cactus plant on the table.

"So, you can feel something come from that cactus?" he said.

"Yes," I said. "As a matter of fact, that's why I bought it. It has a very distinct energy. Why don't you feel for yourself."

He held his hand over the plant.

"I feel something," he said.

He shrugged.

"That's interesting," he commented.

"That's it?" I thought. "'That's interesting.' You don't want to learn more?"

"Dad, let me scan you and see if I can find anything," I said.

Energy radiated outward from the center of his chest. After following the energy strain, I wanted to check the cranial rhythm in his head, since tinnitus usually stemmed from problems in the inner ear. His cranial rhythm was stuck, and unmoving. I waited, until, finally, I perceived some movement.

"Is the ringing in your ears any better, Dad?" I said.

"No, it's still there," he said. "I guess that it didn't do anything..."

In the morning it was nearing 9 AM and my father still hadn't awoken.

"Dad, you better wake up," I whispered. "We're going to be late to your appointment."

"What?!" he exclaimed loudly. "I slept all this time. I haven't slept more than two or three hours in months..."

At the clinic Dr. Rind's medical assistant, Renee, tried to suppress a smile, as she looked back and forth between my father and me.

"I'm struck by your resemblance," she said. "You look like you could be brothers."

Dr. Rind examined my father.

"I think that the source of your tinnitus is the cosmetic dental work that you had done," Dr. Rind said. "Filling in the space between your front teeth has impeded the cranial rhythm. Dental work that results in too close a fit between the teeth can restrict cranial motion by locking the teeth in place and, therefore, restricting the motion at the maxilla..."

After accompanying my father to his appointment at Johns Hopkins and then seeing him off at the airport, I returned to the apartment, and Liz met me at the door.

"I met your father in the hallway yesterday," she said. "Looking into his eyes, it was like gazing into a black hole..."

That night I tossed in bed.

"What's the matter, Michael?" Liz asked.

"I'm not sure," I said. "At Johns Hopkins they put my father through all kinds of tests; but in the end, they weren't able to offer him anything! – Except maybe some advice in case of emergency – And for that, they herded him into a line and charged him an excessive bill."

"And he's suffering," I lamented. "Yet I question how much I care?"

Liz looked at me with an exasperated expression that bordered on disgust.

"Duh!" she responded. "You don't understand the magnitude of your anger. You have to keep looking deeper..."

CHAPTER FIFTY-TWO

Wah invited Albert and me to practice Chi Gong in the backyard of his spacious Potomac home near Great Falls.

"I gain a lot more energy when I perform my Chi Gong exercise outdoors," Albert commented. "Not only am I spinning, but I'm also running as I spin. I go on this way much longer than when I'm indoors."

As I looked out at the fading afternoon light, Wah smiled in my direction.

"What are you thinking about, Mike?" he asked.

"I was thinking about my father," I said. "About the patio barbecues he used to have on nights like these."

I lowered my head.

"Liz tells me that I'm filled with subconscious rage about my father," I confided. "I don't really know what I feel."

"For myself," Albert said, "I have to be near my father as a test to see if I truly forgive and love. If something about being around my dad sends off a trigger of irritation or anxiety, then I know I still have more to work on. I need my father."

"My main hold up," he continued, "is ego and jealousy. The most traumatic event of my life was failing the fourth grade. I was the only oriental to fail the fourth grade. After that, I told myself that I would never fail at something again."

I nodded.

"I remember my first report card," I said. "When my mother saw a couple of B's on it, she wouldn't talk to me."

Albert grimaced, appearing annoyed.

"I don't know," he responded. "I think it's sort of a cop out to blame your parents for your problems."

"You have to live on, Mike," Wah said, "and not be all consumed by the past."

"I'm trying," I said. "But Liz tells me there are things holding me back, and I'm trying to bring them out."

Albert turned his head away in disgust.

"If you live your life in the past this way, then it's a pity," Wah said. "Because, surely, there's much more to life..."

In the yard we practiced Chi Gong. Wah moved in fluid, deliberate steps. It was sunset and his aura shone clearly – surrounding him like a halo, expanding and contracting and enclosing his head in a shimmering light.

Albert, on the other hand, was whirling all around the yard. Watching him, I couldn't detect a definable aura - only the wild, random dissipation of energy, as though he were dangling from the end of a rope, his limbs kicking about...

CHAPTER FIFTY-THREE

"Mike, I had an interesting experience while I was practicing Chi Gong," Liz confided. "I got into a position with my legs crossed, and began knocking on my right leg from the shin to the great toe, and chanting, 'Hate, anger, frustration - leave my body. Hate, anger, frustration - out, out, out.'

"Then, a new chorus started: 'Love, compassion. Don't hate. Love', and it felt like the hatred and frustration I'd been feeling was leaving through my foot."

I nodded.

"Yes, patients have told me about experiences like that," I commented. "After a Bioenergy treatment, they often say that there's a flow of energy that goes out of the body through their feet."

"I think that because many of my organs are blocked," she said, "I feel hate and frustration more often."

She complained of persistent pain in her hips. Scanning her, my hand felt pulled toward her navel, and seemed to be held there, as though being sucked in and out.

"Dantien breathing," I said, astonished.

"What's that?" Liz said.

"It's something that Master Chou has been talking about," I said. "He said that, before we're born, our first source of breathing is through the umbilical cord, near the navel. That's the Dantien point."

"He's been talking about for all these months," I continued "Alluding to it as 'the source of life.' Yet, had it not been for this experience, I would have never understood..."

CHAPTER FIFTY-FOUR

Entering Wah's house, a surge of energy traveled through me, coupled with a feeling of elation and euphoria. Master Chou sat in the living room, looking quiet and cat-like. Paul stood to his left, and when all the chosen assistants had gathered, the Master began to speak.

"The practice of chi gong is a matter of the Master," he said. "The Master creates the chi field. Nevertheless, there are some general guidelines that run through all forms of chi gong."

Several papers were passed out.

The Chi Field.
1. Help people through illness to get to spiritual enlightenment.
2. Always sincerely search for your path.
3. Never use chi gong to betray your conscience or to arrive at ulterior motives.
4. Don't read so much; reading looks at other people's methods of internal searching. Develop your own. You must arrive at your own enlightenment.
5. Intention is key to give the desired message.
6. The chi field is the channel to the universal order.
7. Your chi field is always there; it can be obscured, however, by a negative state of mind. "Clouds might cover the sun, but it is always there; it is just obscured by the clouds."
8. The chi field is a matter of self-cultivation for greater tapping into the universal chi.
9. Regarding helping others via the cultivation of the chi field: "When you are there, I am there."

"In Chi Gong," the Master continued, "we are not looking for tangibles to know that we have helped. In a materialistic society, people need tangibles to start them toward a quest for spirituality. Intellectual acceptance is not enough. A person must open his heart."

Energy technique: "Without touch"
1. Activate intention
2. Recognize that you are a channel to the universal chi (or a representative to serve as a medium).
3. Ask for permission to help another to enhance their gong (This is not a matter of opening channels, as much as it's a matter of enhancing that person's gong via the projection of chi. Blocked and dormant channels are being rejuvenated via the projection of energy to those channels. The instructor is the conduit for helping another person open and restore their channels, and it is chi (energy) from the universal order (universal chi) that facilitates that.
4. Appreciate the permission and ability to help.
5. Don't stand in front of the person.
6. Start with the right-hand, and later become adept with the left.
7. Use no strength. The more relaxed, the better.
8. Afterwards, you will have a sense of joy.
9. Appreciate the other person.
10. Upon completion of chi projection, you will feel your hand rejected, as it seems to bounce off, and you will feel a need to stop. This does not mean that the other person is healed; only that he/she has received as much as they can from you.
11. Do not think about affecting the other person's gong; it is not a matter of opening channels; it is a matter of transmitting energy to enhance that person's gong.
12. Energy transfer will work on everyone.
13. No touching in this technique.
14. Be in a chi gong state, but this should not have to involve any formalities, as the chi gong state can be arrived at spontaneously without any bows.

"Have you truly given your true selves to the gong?" he continued. "In other words, are you truly acting normal? If not, how is the body supposed to know its optimal ability? For the body to function at its highest, it must not be driven by a confused mind. A combination of personal energy and ability to channel the healing energy of the universal is needed."

"Chi Gong requires a serious commitment," he said, "because the capacity for harm is just a great as the capacity for good.

Although most of the time you could be wanting to do good, a change of heart - even for a split second - can unleash a torrent of evil."

"Remember, overcoming the trauma that binds you requires two things - forgiveness and love. Keep in mind, that it is by thinking more about others, and less about ourselves, that we achieve true enlightenment…"

Chi Gong massage technique: "With touch"
1. Put hands on the place where the person is injured.
2. Don't press.
3. Use mindset.
4. Completely intuitive.
5. Use five finger of hand, and let the hand move back-and-forth in a hinge-like manner.
6. Gong will show itself.
7. Maintain a sense of respect. Don't rely on the other person's response as an indicator of your ability; their attitude and mind-set is just as critical a factor as yours in their ability to derive help (i.e., they must be open to you).

"The metal coin pressed to clay leaves an impression. Clay pressed to clay leaves none. One must be firm in his beliefs before he can help others. The missionaries went out, but always stopped teaching sooner or later. When asked what was the problem, they discovered that their error lay in not believing in what they were doing…"

Note: Whether to use touch or non-touch is completely dependent on the needs of the other person. Their need will guide you. Neither technique is more efficient than the other. It just a matter of what the other person needs. It's all intuitive as to the determination of which technique to apply.
Record any revelations you might feel while applying this technique to another.
Don't ever apply these techniques to someone practicing another form of Chi Gong.

"Can a person do Chi Gong and still receive other forms of help? Yes. Would not tell others to quit medications. Medicines are the responsibility of the physician. Would, however, ask the person to get more frequent checkups with his physician to monitor medication needs and changes. One doctor notice that a patient was getting better with chi gong. He told his patient that his meds were not the source of his recovery - as the drugs only obscured the pain - and told him that it was the chi gong that was helping him recover.

"Movement is the way of balance. Have I ever seen someone not advance in Chi Gong and asked him to go elsewhere for help? No. Remember our credo - 'Never give up.' What can help one more than efforts to arrive at the true self and find the way to unlock his body's innate intelligence for the answers to the help himself?

"Do you think that you are smarter than God? Science gives us discoveries that work for everyone. Chi Gong focuses on the individual, relating the uniqueness of his or her experience to find a way to help. How will you be prepared for life in heaven if you haven't manifested it in yourself on earth?

"An appreciation of nature goes hand in hand with being in harmony with the universal chi. The universal chi is everywhere in our lives; Chi Gong helps you receive its healing benefits."

"I am not preparing you for the response of open, thoughtful, good-hearted people," Master Chou concluded. "I am preparing you for what you will face from those who will say that you are stupid, make you the butt of jokes; envy you, ridicule you and make every attempt to deflate and sabotage you.

"Think of yourselves is messengers of life. Think about the messages you have received from the universe. Think about what you wish for? What you would like to request for today? Connect with your old soul what was its original wish, its aspirations. With a sincere heart, request the mercy of the Universal Chi to express yourself and to progress and to be elevated and have a big breakthrough..."

Master Chou announced the end of the day's training. Wah, ever the generous host, said there was a vegan meal awaiting us in the kitchen and we filed over. I filled a plate, then found a solitary place to sit and consume it.

Jennie (one of Master Chou's main assistants) approached me, smiling assuredly.

"Why are you sitting alone, Mike?" she asked.

"I'm just taking it all in," I said. "It feels like we're being imparted a lot of responsibility."

Jennie nodded.

"You have become a 'messenger'," she said. "Master Chou is sending his dharma - To carry on what he teaches you. You are part of him now - To carry on the mission..."

CHAPTER FIFTY-FIVE

Master Chou assembled the new assistants.

"This is the energy endowment," he said. "Before we begin, does anyone have anything they'd like to say?"

I motioned.

"Master Chou, in the past when you've emitted chi, I experienced feelings and questioned whether they were my own?" I said. "I wonder that I can accept this initiation and at the same time pursue my own path?"

"We will be closer after the initiation," he responded, "but that will not take you away from your path."

I considered resisting. A moment later, though, I felt elation, imbued in feeling of energy, large auric fields enveloping my hands…

CHAPTER FIFTY-SIX

At the completion of the induction ceremony, I ventured out alone and walked along a forest path. The Potomac River coursed before me, and I noted some broken glass along the water's edge.

Glass can be smoothed, I thought. It's malleable. But apply too much force and it will fracture and break. The changing process is slow and requires patience and gentility.

Sea shells littered the river bank.

They must be thousands of years old, I told myself. From the time that river emptied into the ocean. Apply sufficient force and the shell will let go of its calcium in the form of chalk, until its form is lost, as it turns to sand. Life provides the force to direct the structure, which, if permitted, can be sustained for years. Form is a combination of substance and life force.

A boulder had broken off from the gorge. At the place where it had fractured were layers of spectacular color.

The color of the stone is always most brilliant beneath the surface, I thought. To get to something beautiful, often you must peel away the layers, go beyond the superficial and find the internal beauty that lay inside...

Returning to the camp, Jennie waved to me.

"Mike, hurry!" she said. "Master Chou is making preparation to perform a healing. He was looking for you..."

Entering the main structure, a tall, older man was sitting on a chair, surrounded by Chi Gong assistants.

"We're going to do this blessing for Mr. Chan," Paul announced.

Jennie directed me closer to Mr. Chan in the center.

"Mr. Chan was in a serious car accident," she whispered, "which resulted in him staying in the hospital for more than a month. Since then, he could not stand with his feet touching each other. He's had surgery to try to help with the pain, soreness, and numbness of his right foot. He took off his sock to show the scar and deformity of the toes. Now, you'll see the 'Without Touch' Chi Gong energy technique as it's supposed to be done."

The Chi Gong assistants seemed to be neatly assembled on each side of Mr. Chan, as though to create human box around him.

"We always have at least one assistant on each side," Jennie explained. "The one in front is to help someone achieve something. The one in back is for support. The one to the left is there for service. The one on the right is also for education. Each will recite four blessings. As they go, you can feel the density of the energy, and the concentration of the energy increase."

Master Chou was standing just beyond his assistants and seemed to concentrate.

"What are you feeling now?" Master Chou asked.

"I feel my foot doesn't hurt anymore," Mr. Chan responded. "I feel like there is almost like a buzz quality there, and it's moving up to my ankle, and gradually moving up to my knee. That's what I feel. I don't know how else to describe it."

"Very good," Master Chou responded. "Your feedback is very important."

Master Chou spoke to the larger group.

"We sincerely request Chi Support to bless Mr. Chan," he said. "Let's pray that Mr. Chan is filled up with universal Chi."

The assistants chanted in Chinese.

"How do you feel now?" Master Chou asked.

"Now, the pain is moving up," Mr. Chan responded. "It feels less swollen. The symptoms are going up to my hip now."

"We are going to do the second round," Master Chou said. "You will have a different feeling after the second round of blessing."

"I bet you wish you could do your own Qi Gong," Jennie whispered. "Bioenergy."

"No," I responded. "I feel very happy to be a part of the group without exerting any individual influence."

Now, the entire group chanted.

"As they say the blessing, breath from your Dantien," Master Chou instructed. "Breathe from that area. Breathe in a ball of energy."

"You don't need to think," Master Chou added. "You just receive. We should be breathing energy into you."

"Now, we all blessed together," Master Chou continued. "We are all connected to the four-sided column of energy. Do you feel the difference? Any particular side feel more dense?"

"During the blessing, in the beginning, I felt numbness and tingling," Mr. Chan said. "Mostly numbness. Now, I'm sore."

"If you feel numb, and you want to move, then move your leg," Master Chou said. "Go ahead and move your leg. Move your foot. Take the energy there and shake it up. And if it feels sore or swollen, tingling, numb, you put energy in the area, bring the blessing to that area and that is what you'll keep."

The chanting continued.

"How do you feel now?" Master Chou asked.

"Everything is unblocked," Mr. Chan said. "Flowing freely. I feel ready to stand up."

The patient stood.

"I feel young!" he called out. "I feel all blessed again. I feel like a new being. I feel like I have a whole brand-new part. Very light. Very warm. Today, I have experienced her chi."

"All who want to receive healing, come forward and pass through the circle," Master Chou cried. "Step forward. Walk through the center. Don't be shy. Go in there. Walk in there. Step into the center. Feel the blessing. Receive the energy. That is a place of healing to occur."

Jennie directed me to the center. Walking through the circle, I became aware of a change – like I was walking in an integrated way that I never had before.

"I'm walking on to two feet!" I exclaimed. "I'm walking balanced on to two feet! Something's happened! I'm walking balanced on to two feet! It's a real source of joy for me, because, with my muscular problems, it's very, very rare that I'll feel balanced like this. The healing really helped me. And I was a mostly passive observer and would not in any way have expected to be physically affected by the healing – But I was! And I had no wish or active desire for any healing during the blessing – But still I acquired healing!"

"Even though you attended the blessing with no wish or intention to request any healing, your mind and spirit were with us," Jennie said. "With your mind clear and no distractions, I believe the Universal Chi heard your inner voice, deep inside, whispering that you needed healing and comfort, and you got that."

"Congratulations!" she exclaimed. "You strongly believed it, and you were embraced by the Universal Chi's blessings when you need them. I know you do, and so do we all."

Tears came to my eyes as a listened, and I tried to keep myself from shaking my head.

"But I don't," I thought. "I don't believe. It just happened..."

CHAPTER FIFTY-SEVEN

Wah invited Liz and me to his home.

"So how are you doing, Michael?" he said. "Are you happy in your new role as a Chi Gong assistant?"

"I'm still not comfortable with the thought of projecting chi," I said. "Serving as a channel for the universal life force is one thing, but projecting it is another. I can't forget the time that Master Chou built that chi field around me, and the feeling of love and elation that I had. It's blown my mind since. It was like he was literally infecting my mind and inserting an emotion that wasn't there."

"Maybe it is there, Mike," Liz commented.

"What do you mean?" Wah asked.

"I have another explanation," she began. "Mike thinks that Master Chou was inserting something. I wonder if the feeling Mike had is just usually so buried inside of him that he can't feel it? At least not until Master Chou gave him a jumpstart by projecting his chi. For a moment, it restored his ability to feel happiness and warmth inside.

"Long ago Mike suppressed that, because he was always too afraid to feel good - His father was going to make a sarcastic remark and reduce a terrific thing he'd done to something trivial and worthless. Then, again, his mother was no better, with her unyielding standards, which accounts for the very reason that she's so miserable all the time..."

We practiced.

"I connected to my inner spirit," Wah said. "I asked it, 'Had Master Chou given me the chi field?' The answer was no, he's simply helped to connect us to the universal chi..."

CHAPTER FIFTY-EIGHT

At a Health Expo near Cleveland Park, Liz and I bumped into Dr. Rind and Renee, and the four of us chatted, then walked about the fair together.

At the Kirlian photography booth, I stood admiring the auras captured in the sample photographs and turned to Dr. Rind.

"How does it work?" I asked.

"It's like a television camera," Rind explained. "The electrons surrounding the person are scattered by an electric current generated by an electric pad under the person's hands, then get caught by the camera over a long, ten-second exposure."

Dr. Rind then generously insisted that all of us have our pictures taken.

Liz's picture was full of white and blue.

"These are the colors of fidelity and spirituality," the photographer explained.

There was a white halo above her head. At her left side was the color green.

"The left side symbolizes what is in your future," said the photographer. "It suggests the entrance of great healing capacities in your future."

"The arc of color over my head is not complete," Liz said.

I looked at her picture, then at the ones on the wall.

"That's right," I said. "In all the other pictures the arch over people's heads is balanced."

I turned to the photographer.

"What does that mean?" I asked.

"It suggests that her future is still uncertain," he answered.

Renee's aura was solid green.

"According to color chart, green is the color of healing," I said. "I guess it's a sign that you're a true healer."

"And, look," Liz said. "On your left side, there's even more green. That means there's even more healing in your future..."

My picture was full of vibrant color, with an arch of greens and yellow and purple and stars.

"You look like the NBC peacock," Dr. Rind laughed.

My heart was purple and on my right side was the color red.

"That means that the outward appearance to others is one who radiates energy," explained the photographer. "On your left side is purple. It symbolizes a spiritual future..."

Blue and white poured forth from Dr. Rind's picture.

"You have a mystical and spiritual nature," said the photographer...

Leaving the photography stand, I turned to Liz.

"I feel happy for Dr. Rind," I confided. "I worry sometimes about his spiritual side - I guess because he reminds me of my father so much."

"I think that it's a testament to our true natures," Liz responded. "That in spite the kind of withholding grounding that Dr. Rind got in his traditional Jewish upbringing, he could still possess such a spiritual aura."

"I wonder if it's because of the work that he does?" I asked. "Whether it's simply the influence of Bioenergy?"

"I don't think so," Liz responded. "It's not by accident that he's a healer who works with Bioenergy..."

CHAPTER FIFTY-NINE

Leaving the Health Expo, Liz and I boarded the Metro. At the next station a man with a limp entered the train. He wore an intense expression, as though every move required intense, concentrated effort. He took a seat some ten feet away (though still in my line of vision) and my leg began feeling warm, then hot, as a feeling of energy collected over my knee.

"Is this interlink?" I thought.

Liz looked at me.

"Is something the matter, Mike?"

"I don't know, Liz," I whispered. "I feel like I'm somehow doing Bioenergy with this man who got in the train."

"Maybe you are," she said.

"But without consciously trying or scanning or following the energy?" I responded, skeptically.

"Perhaps, he doesn't know how to ask you, but still needs your help," she said.

"Well, should I ask him?"

"I don't think so," she said. "Just breath deep, Mike. Let the energy flow through you."

The warmth in my leg finally cooled. When I looked again, the man's expression appeared one of awed relief...

CHAPTER SIXTY

Wah and I had plans to practice Chi Gong at his home. But on receiving me at the door, Wah seemed to stagger.

"Are you alright, Wah?" I asked. "You don't look good."

"I'm having an inner ear problem," he said. "It started yesterday. I've had them before. They usually last a couple of days."

"Can I help?"

Feeling for his cranial rhythm, it was irregular and locked at several points along the skull.

"How long have you had this problem, Wah?" I inquired.

"As long as I can remember," he said. "I had a head injury when I was a child."

The rhythm was slowly surfacing, and I moved from one block to the next. Then, I began to feel dizzy, and a sensation of energy erupted on the right side of my head, just behind my ear.

"Wah, are you feeling anything?" I said.

"Whatever you were doing was helping," he said. "I feel a little better, but I'm still having a problem."

"Where is the problem?" I said.

"Well, before you started, I was feeling it all over my head," he said. "Now, there's just a little left over the right side."

"Where on the right side?" I said.

"In back of my ear," he said.

I staggered back, then looked at him.

"Wah, let's do chi gong," I said.

Entering a chi gong state, a feeling of energy permeated the sides of my head. It was superficial at first, mostly along the scalp. Then, the area behind my right ear erupted again, till the top of my head began to pulsate. Standing upright, I breathed deeply. Finally, the splinter area dissipated, and the buzz passed into a state of clear thinking.

"Wah, I've had an insight," I said. "But first, would you let me try to work on that inner ear problem of yours again?"

Perceiving the energy at the site, I followed it. Slowly, the energy dissipated, until it had fully evaporated from my hand.

"The problem is gone," he told me. "The dizziness. The headache. How did you do that?"

I smiled.

"I think that I understand the relationship of Bioenergy and Chi Gong," I said. "It has to do with serving as a channel for healing. When I treat others using Bioenergy, I permit the universal chi to move through me so as to correct an energy imbalance in another. My capacity to heal relies on my ability to channel the life force; where I'm blocked, I cannot act as an effective channel."

"So, what does that mean?" Wah said. "If you are blocked, then it's just the other person's loss?"

"No, it's the other way around," I responded, spiritedly. "Earlier, when I worked on you, I wasn't quite able to get at your problem. It was because I was blocked the same way you were. I'd also had a head injury as a child and suffered from headaches and dizzy spells. As a result, I couldn't act as a channel for you. But working on you had the effect of bringing that blockage to the surface. It transformed it from something chronic and dormant, to acute and activated – when problems are most amenable to healing.

"So trying to help you, alerted my own body-mind to the blockage. This is the answer to the riddle that I've been searching for… By helping you, you helped me. Don't you see, Wah? All this time I've been fearing that funny 'buzz' I get from some of my patients. I don't need to fear it – Because, really, it's just bringing to the surface my own hidden problems. And with Chi Gong, I can heal those problems as they arise – It's simply a matter of tapping into the Universal Life Force when that happens and reconciling those old wounds."

"Wah, I've found it!" I exclaimed, striking my thighs. "I've found the cure for what ails me! And best of all, my own patients are the ones enabling me to heal these dormant traumas."

"These same patients who I've been shying away from," I concluded, joyous. "It's they who have the most to give me!…"

CHAPTER SIXTY-ONE

My father called, saying he had tickets good for travel anywhere in the world.

"I'm going to give them to you and your brother," he said...

Calling my friend, Ben, I asked for his advice.

"You've danced all over the world," I said. "Which country has the best nature?"

He responded without a moment's hesitation.

"South Africa," he said...

Shortly after, my brother (Joe) and I were on a plane to South Africa...

CHAPTER SIXTY-TWO

Joe had brought his surfboard and wanted to surf the beaches of South Africa. We traveled east to the city of Durban, and while he enjoyed surfing, I visited a local art shop, where I stood admiring some tribal sculpture.

"You like what you see?"

Turning, I saw standing before me a beautiful Indian woman, with strong features, dark sun-drenched skin and lush black hair.

"I'm Pam," she said. "I'm the owner of this shop. This sculpture is made of sandstone. The sculptor lives in Swaziland - a tiny, mountainous country, surrounded by South Africa."

"I like artists," she continued. "I support many throughout Africa. Whenever I find a good sculptor, I collect his works and sell them in my shop."

Another woman entered the shop and called to Pam in demanding fashion.

"I am coming from Cape Town," the woman said in a proper tone. "I hear you sell antique Zulu tribal masks here."

Pam showed her a mask of striking primal beauty.

"You see the marks?" Pam said. "It is said that before a battle, the Zulu warriors put themselves in a deep trance, so that the only way they can come out of it, is by casting the mask off, sometimes throwing it high in the air."

I looked on in awe, imagining being the holder of such a possession.

"I think that $200 is too much," said the woman customer. "Would you take $150?"

Pam politely declined, and the woman said that she'd consider it and come back later.

Pam looked away, despondent.

"In another shop the same quality mask costs five times as much," she said. "She doesn't buy it at the price I gave her because she thinks I'm Indian, and all Indians ask too much and can always be bargained down."

Pam turned to me.

"What do you think of the mask?" she asked.

"I think it's extraordinary," I responded.

"Then, you must take it," she insisted. "I give it to you for $100. I want you to have it because you value it, and even for twice as much, I do not want to see it go to someone like her..."

Small children ran in and out of the shop; Pam greeting them with smiles and lavishing them with treats. She glowed with life, as though it were everywhere around her and touched everything she did.

She asked about my work, and I told her about Dr. Rind's clinic.

"I have difficulty relaxing," she said. "Maybe you would show me one of your techniques?"

"We can try cranial sacral therapy," I said. "Let me show you what I'm doing, Pam. I'm feeling for your cranial rhythm. If you put your hands on each side of mine, you can feel for it through my hands."

The rhythm was locked on the left side. Then, a still point occurred.

"Pam, it looks like I'm picking up on something," I said. "These kinds of things are usually the result of head injury, but it could be anything. Would you mind if I asked your body some questions?"

Counting through the years of her life, "three" produced a twitching along her head.

"Did something happen to you when you were three?" I asked.

Pam's sister had been sitting on the other side of the shop, looking on; now, the two stared at each other.

"How did you know that?" the sister asked, surprised. "When she was three, she fell out of a cart on to an iron rod. She has suffered headaches on that side since."

Shortly after, the cranial rhythm returned, the blockage gone.

"I feel better," Pam said. "Very relaxed, which is all that I really wanted..."

Returning to the hotel, Joe talked about his day of surfing.

"I get out of the water," he began, "and I'm walking down the beach and these guys are like, 'Hey, I see your board. Hey, I can see your style. Where are you from?'

"So, the American kid with the nice surfboard is meeting all the surfers. Come with me down to the beach…"

Meeting Joe on the boardwalk, he was surrounded by several young, blond, tanned men.

"Mike, I met these guys on the beach and told them you do Bioenergy, and they wanted to try it," Joe said.

The first fellow suffered from heartburn. Following a line of energy, it moved downwards from his chest, towards his stomach and outwards.

"Man, my heartburn is gone," he said. "I haven't felt like this in days. This guy is a magician. He's a miracle man…"

"Oh, my knee been hurting," said a second fellow. "Do you think you could take a look at my knee?"

Following the path of energy from his knee, it led me to his shoulder.

"A few years ago, I fell fifteen feet from a balcony," he said. "I landed on my shoulder."

As I continued to follow the energy's path, Robert contorted his body.

"Whoa!" he exclaimed. "I'm perspiring all over."

Finally, the energy was squarely in my hand, and I flicked it away.

"Man, my pain is gone!" he exclaimed. "Let's go surf!…"

A third fellow complained of pain in his jaw; however, when I scanned him, I encountered a shell of energy all around him.

"I don't know what this is?" I said, confused. "I think you need to see a dentist…"

CHAPTER SIXTY-THREE

While Joe continued surfing in Durban, I traveled north to visit several national parks in South Africa and Swaziland.

Returning to Durban about a week later, Joe told me that his surfer friends had asked for me.

"They were saying, 'Your brother is a miracle man. He's a magician. Where is he? We brought all these other mates down. They want to get worked on.' And I said, 'Oh, man, he's off to the national parks.'

Joe said he and they were convinced I could perform miracles.

"When you got that guy's heartburn and then you removed it," he began. "And you felt the energy at the other guy's mouth, and you told him, 'You got to go see the dentist', and he did and the next day he said, 'I got a cavity.' They all told me, 'Your brother... He's incredible.'

"And you'll continue to perform these miracles, because that's who you are. I saw it with my own two eyes. I got to witness it, one, and then, two, I got the corroboration the next day. People don't just say things like that if they're not true and based upon fact. I didn't say, 'My brother is a miracle maker.' No, they had this, and you said, 'Hey, I could try that. I could give it a shot', and then, boom, you were gone. And then the next day, they came up to me and told me.

"So, now, when I tell people what you can do, I'm not just telling them a story based on what you've told me, I'm telling them what I observed and what people then told me! So, if people wanna believe it, believe it. If they don't, they don't. But I know the truth.

"So, keep on doing what you're doing with confidence and that humility you carry and that generosity in your heart. And the good people that you've surround yourself with. And enjoy your life. And know that that's what grandpa Matty and grandma Freida would want. They would want to be able to know that."

Maybe I should stay in South Africa? I responded. Because I don't think Bioenergy will ever be accepted by the medical community in the United States.

"I have a true belief that the miracles are going to continue to be performed until the time that what you do is approved," he responded. "But just like I had to pass the Board to become a lawyer, if they say you have to perform a test to get Bioenergy approved, you'll do it."

"Heed my words, my brother," he concluded. "Stay strong and courageous, as you have always been. It will come to fruition..."

CHAPTER SIXTY-FOUR

My mother called to me sweetly.

"Michael, I want you. Michael."

Then, her tone changed.

"Michael, you asshole, I want you because I want to get better. Michael. You asshole."

It seemed as though she were planning her funeral, with exquisite detail and knowledge of French style. I roamed the house, never finding what I wanted...

Elizabeth moaned, and I awoke from the dream.

"Mom?" I said. "Are you alright?"

She was balled up in pain.

"I'm not your mother," she said, disappointed.

Since returning from South Africa, Liz was having problems of migraine.

"I'm sorry, Liz," I said.

Frustrated, she got up and took a blanket and went into the bathroom. Following her behind the shut door, I found her laying on the cold tile floor.

"You can't sleep here, Liz," I said. "It's no good for you."

"I can't stand the loneliness," she insisted. "Being in so much pain and feeling completely rejected by you."

I led her back to the room.

"Why are you rejecting me?" she demanded.

She sighed, then rested with her head on my chest.

"Your heart seems buried," she said. "It never beats very strong. It stays put behind the walls of your breastbone. The pulses at your feet feel stronger than your heart."

"As stubborn as you are, it doesn't leave a lot of space for divine inspiration or knowing," she continued. "It feels as though you're constantly putting a cap on your ability to feel. It's as though you're afraid of feeling joy because you're too afraid that it's going to be taken away from you - by your father, perhaps, or the worry that he's going to leave you. So rather than chance the pain of that joy being taken away, you take it away yourself - because, at least that's within the bounds of your control, and you don't have to experience it being ripped away from you. But by doing that, you've gypped yourself out of life's joy and happiness..."

Later in the night I awoke to a feeling of agonizing chest pain. Liz lay with her arm draped over my chest. I tried to breathe - but something wouldn't let me.

"Where is it coming from?" I thought. "Bubbles, mother, father, childhood? I don't know..."

"After you went back to sleep," Liz told me, "your body became agitated. You were snorting and panting and making all kinds of anguished sounds. You were talking in your sleep, saying that coming face to face with the pain in your heart, and it was too much for you, and that you needed to turn away and take some time to recover. I felt over you chest. I could feel the bursting forth of your contained heart. It was like it was hammering out the dents in a wrecked car. In my mind I tried to communicate a message, saying, 'It's okay if you need to turn away. Just know that I love you, and that I'm here for you.'

"You stopped snorting and panting then, and a smile came to your lips.

"Your body turned. And, instead of going to the other side of the bed, you moved back to be cradled in my arms..."

CHAPTER SIXTY-FIVE

In this my heart so full of you,
Is a tiny place where ever-present night dwells without stars.
If you will light me a candle and hold my hand,
I will go and see what is there.
Then, maybe, I will feel the warm glow of the bright colors
That dwell,
In the expansive chambers
Where ever-present day enjoys the delights of life
With you in my heart

Liz shared the poem she'd written.

"I had this thought about you while I was doing Chi Gong this morning," Liz said. "Remember we were talking about your heart pain and I thought you might try an opposite approach from what would seem the intellectually logical one? That is, when you have heart pain, instead of recoiling from it, or delving deeper into it to discover or face the source of the pain, or even instead of nursing you crushed heart, what if - sometimes - you tried using it to love, exercising it, teaching it to love, trying out different feelings or aspects of love, just one at a time, slowly, little by little."

"You've said that you tend to get the pains when you're getting love, affection or positive feelings from someone else," she continued. "Perhaps, they're particular loves that you didn't get or were denied as a child and the sudden receiving makes you remember the pain of not getting before.

"So trying to exercise you own ability to love at that point might shift the emotional emphasis from a heart that sees itself as a destabilized victim to one that sees itself as an independent functioning lover of itself, yourself and others - the shift is from a weak position to a strong one..."

CHAPTER SIXTY-SIX

Sponsoring a program for handicapped children, a little boy eating a jelly sandwich made with challah bread took me aside.

"I'm playing on a basketball team now," he said.

"Where I went to high school," I said, "all the best students played on the basketball team. They're probably all rich now."

Then, I thought about my scientific advisor and work at the lab.

"I have to go now," I told the child.

"You're shooting yourself in the foot," he responded...

Awakening from the dream I looked at Elizabeth, still sleeping.

"Liz is sick again," I thought. "She's slowly wasting away. We can't figure out the problem. All the tests are coming back negative. She can't go on living this way."

Just then, Liz awoke and turned to me, smiling.

"What do you like to do most?" she asked.

I shook my head and shrugged.

"What work do you like the most?" she continued.

"Bioenergy," I responded.

She smiled.

"Then, you'll do that..."

CHAPTER SIXTY-SEVEN

Elizabeth's family in Rhode Island were having a family reunion and invited Liz and me to attend. On the way we stopped in New York and visited my aunt and uncle. In the backyard I played soccor with their children.

"How do you like the kids?" my aunt asked.

"I adore your children," I said. "They're extraordinarily good-natured."

I shook my head.

"What fascinates me most is that they aren't vengeful," I continued. "When one accidently hurts another, they don't go after the other. It's something totally alien to me. When I was a kid, I wanted revenge. These kids don't seem to have that…"

Just then, the oldest child, Lanie, played with a balloon behind her mother. When it exploded my aunt jumped, startled.

I was sure that my aunt would be upset and turn on Lanie. Instead, my aunt laughed and cradled Lanie in her arms…

"Mike, it doesn't just come naturally," Elizabeth explained that evening when we were alone. "At the moment that Lanie popped that balloon, your aunt made a conscious choice; she could act with anger, or she could respond with love. She chose the latter. Your problem is that in the home where you grew up, your parents always chose the angry response…"

CHAPTER SIXTY-EIGHT

In the wee hours of the morning, I awoke and went into the kitchen. Not long after, my uncle lumbered in, looking tired and worn out.

"Like some coffee, Michael?" he asked. "How did you sleep?"

"Not so good," I said. "I had a nightmare."

He kept his gaze averted.

"What about?" he asked.

I leaned back.

"I was leading a squadron of the Israeli secret service," I began. "Shots had been fired within the headquarters, and I was assigned to make sure that everything was in order.

"My men and I were going from command post to command post, I was going from command post to command post. Outside of headquarters it was a bright and shiny, beautiful day, with light like I remember in Tel Aviv or New York. I felt assured and confident.

"But back at headquarters, we were alerted that more shots had been fired. Inside, four bullet tracts - side-by-side - had been left in a table, probably shot from below.

"Then, something caught my eye. It was an oriental man. I'd seen earlier in the day, but, now, he looked different, as though he'd suddenly acquired some added girth about the abdomen and chest.

"'That's strange,' I thought.

"But I let the observation go, thinking it was sad and strange that he'd gained the weight somehow, but that I had to keep on moving.

"My men and I were seated in an office, behind a closed glass door in an underground bunker underground when, suddenly, the lights went out. I didn't give it much thought, at first - I figured it was an electrical outage, and they'd come back on again.

"Then, behind the glass, a figure appeared outside the door.

"'I can't reach my gun,' I told the others. 'Have yours ready.'

"The shadowy figure shattered the glass, and my men emptied the chambers of their weapons into his body. When the gun fire ceased and the smoke cleared, the stranger was still standing and slowly made his way towards us. It was the oriental man, and what I had let pass for added girth was, in actuality, a bullet proof vest. Then, one-by-one, he shot each of us from point-blank range.

"The next thing that I remember, my men and I were working behind the counter of a butcher shop. Officials from headquarters pulled me aside and implored me to come back to work. I ripped open my shirt – the wound still fresh.

"'Look at me!' I told them. 'What can a man with a hole in his chest possibly do?!'"

I shook my head.

"Liz says that my dreams are impossible to interpret," I asserted. "'They're just too weird,' she says."

"No, wait a minute," my uncle intoned gently. "Let's think about it. Did you recognize any of the people in the dream?"

"I think, maybe, the oriental man was my friend, Wah Lee. But, otherwise, no, I didn't recognize anyone."

He stood stirring the cream into his coffee.

"What does 'Israel' represent?" he asked, reflectively. "It's the Jewish state. In a sense it's like home. A squadron is your primary unit within an organization – the members are like family. Guns - these are instruments to inflict pain. Being shot upon - that's fear and danger. People in a bunker - a place of vulnerability. The man with the bullet-proof vest - he's someone who can hurt you. The butcher shop - that's a place where things are cut on, like an operating room. Opening your shirt - You're saying that you're hurt, and you can't help others as long as you're hurting."

"You say that you don't recognize any of the people in the dream," he continued. "That might symbolize your putting your life on the line for strangers. I mean, let's face it, you've always put others first..."

CHAPTER SIXTY-NINE

Arriving at the family home in Providence, we were greeted by the members of Liz's family. In the backyard, Liz introduced me to her brother, Teddy, who was tending the garden, and looked weak and depleted.

"My bronchitis has come back," he explained. "I was sick all night."

"Teddy, if it's alright, may I work on you?" I asked.

Scanning his chest, the energy from his heart chakra felt weak. Following the strain pattern, something unusual happened, as the energy evaporated all at once. Feeling over his chest again, this time the energy rain down from his heart, descending like flowing arcing waterfalls into the ground.

"I feel better," he said, "like there's been a break in the fever that I've had all week long. I'd been looking into your eyes while you worked on me - I felt like I could see into your life. I thought that I saw where you lived. It looked like one large room - maybe a studio apartment - with dark floors, probably wood, and lots of plants. There was a woman - lover, friend, companion - who loved you, but you couldn't be sure that you loved her."

"As a matter of fact, I do live in an efficiency apartment," I said, "with hard wood floors that I like to dance on. And Elizabeth has filled the place with plants."

"You're a warm person," he said. "I'm glad my sister has a friend like you."

Teddy left for a friend's wedding. Liz smiled.

"I felt sure that something good would happen when I got you and Teddy together," she said. "Teddy is someone who can help you move through your fear…"

CHAPTER SEVENTY

Teddy came by the following day.

"How is your bronchitis?" I asked.

"I've mostly recovered," he said. "But what's really bothering me now is my leg... I twisted my back a year ago while digging up a large rock in the backyard, and have had sciatic nerve problems ever since."

"Can I work on you again?"

Scanning his head, I felt an energy reach out to me. Slowly, I moved back, but our energies were still entwined.

"I feel much better," he said. "I'm breathing easier, and the leg pain is gone."

"I thought that I could see into your mind again," he continued. "I saw a desk - long and flat and white - with a curled object on it, perhaps a lamp."

"That's right," I said. "Your sister made that desk for me. She constructed it out of a door."

As Teddy drove off, my back underwent a kind of shifting. It felt as though I were standing on my own two feet for the first time, and walking was an entirely new experience...

"You need Teddy," Liz said, "because you've never had a warm male role model before..."

CHAPTER SEVENTY-ONE

"What I'm afraid of," I confided to Teddy, "is life's uncertainties... What if I get into a car wreck? What if my boss doesn't like me? What if I lose my job? What then?"

Teddy hesitated.

"My attitude is that I can do anything as long as the prospects are good, and I'm careful, I don't have to surround myself with 'What ifs?'" he responded.

He broke off.

"While you were working on me yesterday," he continued. "I'd been directing my intention on you, shining a white healing light all through your spine."

"It helped!" I replied, spiritedly. "Afterward, it felt like I was walking balanced for the first time."

Teddy was quiet.

"When I work with people, I want to direct my energies at getting them better," he said. "With you, it's different... You want to help people get through it – You open the way for them to do it by themselves..."

CHAPTER SEVENTY-TWO

In the morning Teddy came to the house.

"Mike, you want me to show you how to ride a motorcycle?"

I had problems taking off.

"You have to commit to it," he said. "You're treating it with too much trepidation. You have to commit. Have you ridden one before?"

"Once," I said. "My father had a motorcycle, and I asked him if he could teach me ride it. 'Oh, okay,' he said. 'First, you take you hand off the clutch.' 'Where's the clutch, Dad?' I asked. 'You don't know where the clutch is?!' he screamed. 'No, I don't, Dad,' I said. 'Well, it's over here. Then, you give it some acceleration.' 'How do I do that, Dad?' 'You don't know how to use the accelerator!...'

"Finally, I rode off, and it wasn't long before I realized I didn't know how to stop. Even when I took my hand off the accelerator, the motorcycle kept going forward. I was out of control. I went off the road, but the motorcycle kept accelerating. I was on a lot, and moving closer and closer to a brick wall in front of me, till, finally, I jumped off. I went rolling over and over. I was bleeding from cuts and scrapes everywhere. My father comes running up behind me. 'Look what you've done to my bike,' he says."

Teddy was quiet, and I followed him as he walked to the garage.

"You should have seen the things that we pulled out of this place after our father died," he said. "Driver's licenses, keys, money, tapes, belts, women's clothing. Our father was a mad man. He would scream. One time he accused me of stealing his tools. In reality, he'd been stealing from me.

"He'd slap me in the face when I didn't learn fast enough. Afterwards, I wasn't able to progress in school. They diagnosed me

131

with dyslexia, and put me in a special school. To this day I still can't read..."

Inside, Lena had prepared brunch.

"I had it tough with my husband," she said, triumphant. "And even tougher with my father before that. But, through it all, it helped me to realize the most important thing of all... Self-actualization."

"Mike's mother and father might not have had much of a marriage," she continued, "but, through it all, they produced someone like Mike. You never know how things might turn out and what good will happen..."

CHAPTER SEVENTY-THREE

Liz had an appointment with a naturopathic physician in Connecticut. In the patio of his modest and pleasant home office, he quietly examined her, then recommended several healing remedies...

"So, what did you think of the doctor?" she asked.

"I thought he was very nice," I said. "I think he's someone who can help you."

"Why don't you become a naturopath?" she said. "It's a gentle approach. You won't hurt your patients with naturopathic and homeopathic remedies. You don't want to prescribe drugs. You won't have to worry about side effects."

"I don't know, Liz," I said. "How would I get into naturopathic school? I don't have money. My health is bad. I'm worried about you. What will I do with my past education? If I went a different path, it would be worthless to me now."

"Well, look on the bright side," she said. "Your health is getting better. You have a better idea of where you're going. You're kind, intelligent, sincere and caring. You've always done well before."

She looked out.

"I think that I have to be here for a while," she said. "I need to be with my family now. I hate the idea of not being with you, but going back to DC is terrible for my health. Between the environment and the people, I'm being murdered. I have to stay here..."

CHAPTER SEVENTY-FOUR

After helping Liz re-locate, she followed me to my car.

"I don't want you to get into any trouble," she said. "The plan is to finish your PhD. After that, who knows? I'll stay in Providence with my mom."

Teddy pulled up on his motorcycle.

"I wanted to say goodbye," he said.

He smiled, but looked thinner, and said he hadn't been eating well. I was happy to see him and tears welled up in my eyes.

"Can I work on your stomach?" I asked.

Scanning him, the energy from his heart chakra was full and healthy, but it felt like a void existed at the stomach. Following the energy outward, it ultimately flowed with such force that it moved through my arm, till splashing out from my elbow.

Teddy put up his hands.

"You have good energy," he said. "Your aura feels cool and balanced."

He looked at me, as though peering into my soul. I wanted to tell him to take care of Liz, but couldn't bring myself to get the words out.

He rode off.

Elizabeth stood beside me.

"Remember, Michael," she said. "There are some people who belong to the world. You're one of those people. Others will hate you, because they want to be like you. Your journey has just begun..."

ABOUT THE AUTHOR

Michael Yanuck, M.D., Ph.D. is a physician-scientist
whose groundbreaking research at the National Institutes of
Health (NIH) was the basis for a FDA-approved vaccine for cancer
that ushered in the science of Neoantigen Tumor Immunotherapy
now used to fight cancer worldwide. Following a traumatic leg injury,
he trained in Bioenergy, introduced energy medicine approaches at
the National Institute of Complementary and Integrative Health,
and worked with Chi Gong Masters who were part of President
Clinton's Executive Committee on Alternative Medicine.
Now, a Professor of Medicine, he leads efforts to
combat the opioid crisis and advance integrative
therapies for the treatment of pain.